Primary Progressive
Multiple Sclerosis

The general resources in Appendix 2 and references within individual
chapters are posted on the websites of the National Multiple
Sclerosis Society at www.nationalmssociety.org/ppms, the Multiple
Sclerosis Association of America at www.msassociation.org/ppms,
and DiaMedica Publishing at http://www.diamedicapub.com/
primary-progressive-multiple-sclerosis/ppms-book-resources/. The
posted version is an "active" PDF that that can be easily downloaded
to your own computer. It is formatted so that clicking on a link will
take you directly to sites on the Internet.

Primary Progressive
Multiple Sclerosis

What You Need to Know

Nancy J. Holland, Ed.D.

Jack S. Burks, M.D.

Diana M. Schneider, Ph.D.

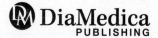
DiaMedica PUBLISHING

Library of Congress Cataloging-in-Publication Data on file.

DiaMedica titles are available for bulk purchase, special promotions, and premiums. For more information please contact us by telephone at (212) 752-2098 or visit our website: www.diamedicapub.com.

Book design: TypeWriting
Cover design: Steven Pisano

ISBN: 978-0-9823219-0-4

Disclaimer
The information in this book is not intended as a substitute for medical or other professional advice. The reader is encouraged to consult his or her physician, or other health care professional about all health matters that might require professional diagnosis and/or medical attention.

Acknowledgments

We are grateful to the many individuals who provided expert reviews of this book:

From the National Multiple Sclerosis Society: Nancy Law, Executive Vice President, Programs and Services; Dorothy Northrop, M.S.W., A.C.S.W., Vice President, Research and Clinical Operations; Rosalind Kalb, Ph.D., Vice President, Professional Resource Center; Nicholas LaRocca, Ph.D., Vice President, Health Care Delivery and Policy Research; and Patricia O'Looney, Vice President of Biomedical Research.

From the Multiple Sclerosis Association of America: Susan Wells Courtney, Senior Writer & Creative Director; Robert Rapp, M.P.A., Vice President of Programs & Partnerships; and Andrea L. Griesé, Vice President of Communications & Marketing.

And our respected colleagues: Pat Bednarik, M.S., CCC-SLP, MSCS; Sharon Dodge; John Fowler, J.D.; Andrew D. Goodman, M.D.; Miriam Franco, Ph.D.; Don Fredette, Adaptive Equipment Specialist; and Patricia G. Provance, P.T., MSCS.

We would especially like to thank the individuals who helped in the development of the accompanying DVD and whose comments appear throughout the book, helping to bring to the reader the perspective of others living and coping with PPMS: Tom Holtakers, a retired physical therapist in Rochester, Minnesota, who has had PPMS since 1972; Kathy Kemph, who has lived with PPMS since the early 1990s; her husband Bob Kemph; Shelley Peterman Schwarz, who lives in Madison, Wisconsin, and is a professional writer and speaker about a wide variety of disability-related issues; her husband Dave Schwarz; and Jason DaSilva, a filmmaker in his 20s who lives in New York City.

Dedication

We dedicate this book to Phyllis Wiesel-Levison, B.S., R.N., Pamela F. Cavallo, M.S.W., A.C.S.W., Linda A. Morgante, M.S.N., R.N., C.R.R.N., and Nancy Cobble, M.D., pioneers in the comprehensive care of individuals with MS and their families; and to everyone living with and affected by primary progressive multiple sclerosis.

If you purchased a copy of this book without a DVD prepared by the National Multiple Sclerosis Society, please call 1-800-FIGHT-MS to request a copy.

Contents

PART III: QUALITY OF LIFE: HAPPINESS IS
A STATE OF MIND, NOT OF HEALTH

PART IV: APPENDICES

Preface

This book was developed as a logical outgrowth of the realization that, despite the advances in therapy that have changed the lives of people with the relapsing forms of multiple sclerosis (MS), little has changed for people with primary progressive MS (PPMS). People with this progressive-from-onset form of MS often experience severe and unremitting symptoms, and they have a higher general level of disability than do people with relapsing remitting MS (RRMS) or secondary progressive MS (SPMS), a later stage following relapsing-remitting disease.

Although major advances have been made in delaying or preventing progression for the relapsing forms of MS, to date little progress has been made in controlling the disease process in PPMS. Treatment strategies are largely focused on managing the symptoms of the disease, rehabilitation strategies, and providing counseling and other forms of psychosocial support.

Primary Progressive Multiple Sclerosis: What You Need to Know is part of a major joint undertaking by the National Multiple Sclerosis Society and the Multiple Sclerosis Association of America to help meet the wide range of needs experienced by people with PPMS, their families, and their health care providers. In addition to pharmacologic and other types of symptom management, it discusses ongoing supportive care from nurses, physicians, occupational and physical therapists, and other specialists to address the wide variety of physical and emotional issues that people with PPMS and their families experience while living with a steadily progressive disease.

Early chapters discuss the characteristics of PPMS, how it is diagnosed, and the state of research and clinical trials for the primary progressive forms of MS, and provide an overview of treatment. Later chapters deal with specific issues of critical importance to people with the disease and family members: symptoms and their management, maintaining wellness in the presence of disease, and family, social, and economic issues.

Because we want the book to be used in part as a "jumping off" place in your journey to learn more about PPMS, we have provided references to additional information throughout the text. In addition, the detailed resources in Appendix 2 will lead you to more in-depth information on any topic.

Nancy J. Holland, Ed.D.
Jack S. Burks, M.D.
Diana M. Schneider, Ph.D.
September 2009

Foreword from the National Multiple Sclerosis Society

The National MS Society is a collective of passionate individuals who want to do something about multiple sclerosis *now*—to move together toward a world free of MS. It is a privilege for me to serve as a leader in this movement.

I meet many people with MS in my travels as president and CEO of the Society, and I have heard time and again from people with primary progressive MS about their frustrations. Since 85 percent of people who have MS are initially diagnosed with a relapsing form of the disease, and since all of the currently available treatments have also been approved primarily for use in relapsing disease, it is no wonder that people with a primary progressive course have often felt forgotten and neglected.

I want all of you who live with PPMS to know your voices are heard—and that we at the Society have shared your frustrations about the lack of information available about PPMS. I hope that this publication and companion DVD will begin a new era. We at the National MS Society are committed to learning more about PPMS: who it affects and why, how it might be treated, and what strategies will best mitigate its impact on quality of life. We are committed to research that will help us to understand why MS progresses and how to stop it in its tracks. We are committed to supporting those who live with all forms of the disease, through our 50-state network of chapter programs and services.

We are grateful to our pharmaceutical partner, Genentech, whose interests and sponsorship have helped us to jump-start these initiatives focused on PPMS. Thanks also to our friends at the Multiple Sclerosis Association of America for their collaboration on this initiative.

Joyce Nelson
Chief Executive Officer
National Multiple Sclerosis Society

Foreword from the Multiple Sclerosis Association of America

I am proud of the Multiple Sclerosis Association of America's (MSAA) collaboration with the National Multiple Sclerosis Society to address the very real challenges faced by people with primary progressive (PPMS). MSAA's focus has always been on providing information and services that make tangible and meaningful differences in the lives of individuals affected by MS, including those with PPMS.

Co-authored by MSAA's Chief Medical Officer Dr. Jack Burks, Dr. Nancy Holland representing the National MS Society, and Dr. Diana M. Schneider, this book is a significant contribution to our understanding of PPMS. Most importantly, it provides useful information and resources to help individuals with PPMS maintain their highest possible quality of life.

Primary Progressive Multiple Sclerosis: What You Need to Know addresses the physical, emotional, and social impact of this less common form of MS. It also provides clear explanations of how MS affects the body's immune and central nervous systems, along with encouraging details about ongoing research and hope for the future. This book will prove to be a valuable resource for those with PPMS, their carepartners, family members, and health care professionals.

While we await an approved treatment for PPMS, and ultimately a cure for MS, MSAA will continue to passionately fulfill its mission to "enrich the quality of life for everyone affected by multiple sclerosis." We accomplish our mission by providing vital programs and services to the MS community, such as Helpline support, printed and online information, equipment distribution, MRI assistance, and educational programs of the highest quality. We invite everyone to take advantage of these useful resources, many of which are noted throughout the book.

Douglas G. Franklin
President and CEO
Multiple Sclerosis Association of America
and
President, MS Coalition

About the Authors

Nancy J. Holland, Ed.D., R.N. was with the National Multiple Sclerosis Society for twenty-one years. As vice president of clinical programs, she was responsible for the Society's national professional education programs for health care providers. She was one of the first nurses to specialize in the care of people with MS in the comprehensive care setting, and is a founding member of the International Organization of MS Nurses. She is the author or co-author of more than 70 MS-related publications, including the books *Multiple Sclerosis for Dummies*; *Multiple Sclerosis: A Self-Care Guide to Wellness*; *Multiple Sclerosis: A Guide for the Newly Diagnosed*; and *Comprehensive Nursing Care in Multiple Sclerosis*.

Jack Burks, M.D. is a neurologist who specializes in multiple sclerosis. He is chief medical officer of the Multiple Sclerosis Association of America; director of program development for the MS Comprehensive Care Center at Holy Name Hospital in Teaneck, New Jersey; and president of Burks & Associates Health Care & Research Consulting Group. He was a founder and president of one of the nation's first comprehensive multiple sclerosis centers, the Rocky Mountain MS Center in Denver. Dr. Burks has served on the boards of directors of the American Academy of Neurology, the American Society of Neurorehabilitation, and the Consortium of Multiple Sclerosis Centers, and he is a member of the National Clinical Advisory Board of the National Multiple

Sclerosis Society. He has edited two textbooks of multiple sclerosis management, including *Multiple Sclerosis: Diagnosis, Medical Management and Rehabilitation*, and published numerous scientific articles and reviews, as well as consulting with professionals and patients in more than forty countries.

Diana M. Schneider, Ph.D. originally trained as a neurochemist. She is president and publisher of DiaMedica, which specializes in books focused on a wide range of health-related topics. As founder and publisher of Demos Medical Publishing, she developed an extensive list of books covering a wide range of issues relating to multiple sclerosis, and is currently on the board of the Multiple Sclerosis Quarterly Report and is a member of the Consortium of Multiple Sclerosis Centers. Dr. Schneider has a particular interest in primary progressive MS because her family has been living with the disease for nearly 25 years.

Introduction

Despite the many publications available about multiple sclerosis (MS), a book dedicated to the specific needs of people with primary progressive multiple sclerosis (PPMS) has not been available.

Even when "progressive" MS has been discussed, PPMS has not been adequately distinguished from secondary progressive MS (SPMS). Although the management of symptoms is similar, the disease courses are very different in terms of how they affect peoples' lives. PPMS usually begins after age 40 and has an unremitting course from onset, whereas SPMS develops in people who have previously had the relapsing form of MS, which usually began when they were young adults.

Beginning in the early 1990s, *disease modifying therapies* (DMTs) changed the prognosis of MS for people with relapsing remitting MS (RRMS), and have slowed the transition to SPMS for many individuals. However, people whose disease is progressive from onset have had little hope of relief. They have often been told that little can be done for them. This form of MS is associated with severe and unrelenting symptoms, and people with PPMS often live without the comfort of knowing that an effective therapy is available. However, recent discoveries may change this outlook in the future.

Some people with PPMS refer to their disease as the "orphan" of the MS world. Their attitude is often one of resignation and hopelessness. They believe—with good reason—that most of the attention is directed toward RRMS because of the availability of DMTs, and they are concerned about the relative lack (until recently) of research on PPMS. In part, this lack of treatment has been due to the fact that existing therapies target the inflammatory process that is the primary component of relapsing forms of MS; the primary progressive form of MS, however, involves from its onset neuronal *atrophy*—a loss of neurons that is not necessarily the result of an inflammatory process (also referred to as *neurodegeneration*) and that does not respond to current anti-inflammatory therapies. When inflammation is present, it does not appear to be of the same type as seen in relapsing forms of the disease. This dearth of treatment for PPMS also reflects the difficulty of doing clinical trials with a disease that has a long time course and that lacks easily measurable changes, such as a decline in relapse rate, as well as the much smaller number of people with PPMS versus relapsing forms. This material is discussed in greater detail in Chapter 3.

> *There are positives to having primary progressive MS versus other kinds of MS. You're not going to have a day when you all of a sudden just get up and you can't walk or you can't see. But you're also not going to get a remission either.* — Jason

People with PPMS have a wide range of needs. In addition to pharmacologic and other types of symptom management, they need ongoing therapy and management strategies to make sure that they can take advantage of their existing strengths. This requires supportive care from nurses, physicians, occupational and physical therapists, psychologists, speech and language therapists, and other specialists to address the wide variety of physical and emotional issues that they and their families experience.

The National MS Society and the MS Association of America play major roles in providing information and support for everyone affected by MS. Realizing that this segment of the MS population has had gaps in service, these two organizations, with an educational grant from

Genentech, jointly undertook a major analysis of the available data about people with PPMS and their support needs, with the goal of developing programs to meet these needs.

They began by analyzing existing statistical information about PPMS, using the patient databases of three organizations: The Sonya Slifka Longitudinal Multiple Sclerosis Study, sponsored by the National MS Society; the MS Association of America's 2005–2006 Comprehensive Client Needs Assessment; and the extensive database of the Consortium of MS Centers' North American Research Committee on Multiple Sclerosis (NARCOMS).

To help guide the development of strategic planning and programs, this information was further refined in a series of online discussion groups, which included adults with PPMS and family caregivers, MS specialist neurologists, MS nurses, and psychologists and licensed social workers. Current resources were evaluated, as well as what is currently known by the scientific community.

This was followed by a conference, held in Dallas, Texas, in February 2008, the objective of which was to analyze the data derived from the databases and focus groups and use this information as a basis to recommend programs and resources to address the unmet needs of those with PPMS and their families. Gaps in research were also identified and addressed.

Most people with MS have the relapsing-remitting course, and all of the drugs and all of the treatments tend to be focused on them. The 10 percent or so of us with PPMS have a disease that's called multiple sclerosis but doesn't act the way it does for others. We're like orphans; there's not a lot out there for us.
— Tom

The Characteristics of PPMS

The three databases and the discussion groups indicate the following characteristics of the PPMS population:

▶ Approximately 10 percent of people with MS have PPMS.

▶ The onset of symptoms in people with PPMS tends to occur later than in those with RRMS. They also tend to be older as a group.

▶ A higher proportion of men are affected with PPMS—approximately 50 percent as compared to the 25–35 percent of men in the general MS population.

▶ As a group, people with PPMS tend to be more disabled than those with RRMS or SPMS. They are more likely to be unable to walk; are more likely to need help with activities of daily living, such as dressing or bathing; and they require more home assistance.

▶ People with PPMS are less likely to be working than those with RRMS, and they have lower family incomes. They are also more likely (67 percent) to be on Social Security Disability Insurance (SSDI) than those with RRMS (41 percent) or SPMS (62 percent).

▶ Although there are no differences between people with the progressive and relapsing forms of MS on mental health scales, there *is* a significant difference in attitude toward the disease. People with RRMS live with constant anxiety about new attacks. In contrast, people with PPMS might have less anxiety, but tend to feel a sense of hopelessness and a degree of resignation based on the lack of effective therapies. They have a significantly lower belief in their ability to control their disease and function with it than do those with RRMS.

These observations provided important information about what support services people with PPMS and their families need, and they form the basis for the content of this book. These areas of need include:

▶ The lack of effective therapies and the extent of advanced disease make it critical to provide effective symptom management, as well as to address issues of wellness and the maintenance of optimal health and quality of life in the presence of PPMS.

▶ People with PPMS are likely to need significant assistance in areas such as assistive technology, rehabilitation, psychosocial support, and home and vehicle modifications. In this context, the term *rehabilitation* means taking advantage of what abilities remain, rather than focusing on what has been lost. It will help people with PPMS to relearn skills and find new ways of doing things. It often focuses on such areas as physical therapy to help increase strength, mobility, and fitness, and occupational therapy to help with daily activities such as bathing and cooking.

▶ People with PPMS and their families need information about a wide range of nonmedical issues that are part of living with PPMS, such as employment, insurance, disability benefits, transportation, and adapted recreation.

▶ Individuals with PPMS and their families also need assistance in obtaining financial aid for assistive equipment, home care, adult day programs, housing options, and nursing home care.

▶ People who are working, and who want to continue working as long as possible, need information and assistance with issues such as work accommodations.

▶ PPMS affects the entire family, and family dynamics often undergo significant changes. Family support systems are needed to help face these challenges.

▶ When PPMS involves a significant degree of disability, family members—especially spouses—may find themselves taking on the role of caregiver. It is important that they be supported in a variety of ways to help maintain the family unit and relationships, and that "caregiver burnout" be avoided.

ASSESSMENT AND MANAGEMENT OF NEEDS FOR PEOPLE WITH PPMS

While discussing areas of need, it is important to realize that they are all intertwined. The onset of new symptoms or worsening of existing ones can have serious consequences in many nonmedical areas, ranging from interpersonal and family relationships to economic issues such as employment. Conversely, improvements in symptom control or psychosocial support can contribute to general well-being, as well as improve relationships, the ability to continue working, and other practical issues.

> I found myself in what I call "Groundhog Day Syndrome": where I'd wake up every morning lamenting about what I used to be able to do and what I've lost and, oh, woe is me, I have MS. I'd kind of moan and groan in my own world. I was stuck . . . just focusing on my problem day after day after day. I got nowhere. I started to break out of that by focusing on my future rather than my past.
> — Tom

The analyses and discussions held under the auspices of the National MS Society and the MS Association of America identified a number of broad areas in need of improvement. These included medical management, the management of mental health and emotional issues, quality-of-life needs, family and caregiver support, and education and support for health care providers. A recurring theme was the lack of information on PPMS for everyone concerned—patients, family, and health care professionals.

The task force recommended that more printed materials should be developed for people with PPMS and their families, including information that can be given out at the time of diagnosis. This book was developed to help everyone diagnosed with PPMS—as well as their families and caregivers—better understand the disease and how it can be managed. Additionally, all existing educational materials are being reviewed, updated, and made available in a clearly identifiable place on both the National MS Society and the MS Association of America websites. Many of these suggestions have already been implemented by both organizations, while others are works in progress.

1

What Is Primary Progressive Multiple Sclerosis and How Is It Diagnosed?

The central nervous system (CNS) contains billions of nerve cells called *neurons,* which communicate messages to the rest of the body and control all bodily functions by sending electrical messages along their *axons.* Axons can be likened to electrical wires and—just like them—they require insulation. This insulation is called *myelin.* The disease process in multiple sclerosis (MS) involves damage to the myelin—in a process called *demyelination*—and also damage to the axons themselves because of the loss of their protective coating. When this happens, these electrical messages either get through slowly or not at all.

WHAT CAUSES MULTIPLE SCLEROSIS?

Although it is not yet clear what causes MS, three factors seem to play a role: the immune system, genetics, and environment.

The Immune System

Most researchers believe that MS is an *autoimmune* disease. Some evidence suggests that it might be triggered by a common virus and that certain people are more susceptible to developing MS because of genetic factors. MS is believed to occur in genetically susceptible indi-

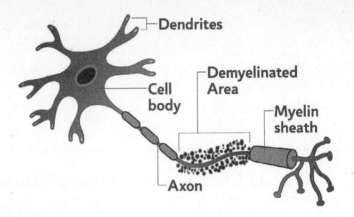

DEMYELINATED NEURON

viduals who come into contact with some infectious trigger(s) in the environment. This exposure likely occurs in childhood, years before clinical symptoms appear. Many triggers, viruses, and bacteria have been studied, but we still do not know the culprit(s). Other studies have looked at diet, vitamin D/sunlight exposure, and toxin exposure. The immune system is discussed in more detail in Chapter 3.

Genetics

Multiple sclerosis is not an inherited disease, in the sense that it is not passed directly from parents to children. However, close relatives do have an increased risk of developing MS, most probably because they inherit the same genes that code for proteins in the immune system that predispose them to the disease. The risk of MS when a parent has the disease is approximately 3 percent, meaning that if you take a hundred individuals with MS, and you look at one child from each person, only three of these 100 children will develop MS at some point during their lives. If you compare this to the risk in the general population which is about one in a thousand, the risk for children with MS is approximately 30-40 times that of the general population risk. Therefore, the true effect of the genetics may not be a large risk, but there is definitely an increase in risk for children. Nonidentical twins of a person diagnosed with MS are affected about 5 percent of the time. Despite the fact that they have an identical genetic makeup, identical twins of people with MS only develop the disease about one-third of the time. The genetic data have not been broken out by disease course, so we do not know whether these statistics are identical for primary progressive MS (PPMS) and MS in general. We also know that when one autoimmune disease is present in a family, there is an increased risk to develop others.

The Environment

Why, even with identical genes, don't most or all identical twins of people who develop MS also develop the disease? The percentages might reflect the role of environmental exposure. A great deal of technical data show the effects of such factors as exposure to specific viruses, geographic latitude, or the age when people move from one climate to another as affecting the development of the disease. Despite this, research has not yet identified what environmental factors are involved in developing MS in the presence of a specific genetic susceptibility, or how they might interact.

THE FOUR COURSES OF MULTIPLE SCLEROSIS

Relapsing Remitting Multiple Sclerosis

Approximately 85–90 percent of all people with MS are diagnosed with relapsing remitting MS (RRMS) at the time of diagnosis. People have *relapses*, also called *exacerbations* or *attacks*. These are followed by periods of full or partial recovery, called *remissions*, during which the disease does not become worse.

> When I was diagnosed, they used the terms exacerbating remitting or chronic progressive. What I noticed was that other people with MS were describing their exacerbations. I wasn't having big flare-ups where I was totally paralyzed one day and walking around the next. So, I realized that there was something different about my MS.
> — Tom

Secondary Progressive Multiple Sclerosis

The term *secondary progressive* MS (SPMS) reflects the fact that it is a later stage of MS that begins as RRMS and then changes to a progressive course. In this stage, remissions become fewer, and the disease steadily progresses. If and when attacks occur, there is little recovery afterwards. Without disease modifying therapy (DMT), approximately 50 percent of people with RRMS will develop SPMS within 10–15 years and as many as 90 percent within 20 years.

Progressive Relapsing Multiple Sclerosis

Progressive relapsing MS (PRMS) is the least common form of MS, occurring in approximately 5 percent of people with the disease. Similar to those with PPMS, people with PRMS experience disease progression from the very beginning, but they also experience occasional *relapses*. Because PRMS is progressive from onset, a doctor might initially diagnose PPMS and then change the diagnosis to PRMS when relapses occur. During these relapses, a person is likely to experience new symptoms or a sudden worsening of previous ones that lasts for days to months and then gradually subsides.

Because people with PRMS may respond to the DMTs used for relapsing remitting disease, many neurologists recommend a DMT for progressive patients who experience relapses.

I had a strange form of MS. It got worse every single day. I couldn't understand why I was never stable. I never got anything back. If I lost it, it stayed lost.
— Shelley

Primary Progressive Multiple Sclerosis

Primary progressive MS is slowly progressive from the beginning, without the attacks that characterize the relapsing-remitting form of MS, occuring in approximately 10 percent of people with the disease. It is characterized by a higher incidence of spinal cord disease as compared to symptoms such as the vision or sensory difficulties that are commonly seen in RRMS. PPMS tends to begin later in life, usually after age 40.

WHAT IS PPMS?

The diagnosis of PPMS used to take a long time—sometimes years—because it was based on a clinical pattern that might only become apparent over time. If you were diagnosed with MS some years ago, this might apply to you. Many people diagnosed with "chronic progressive MS" have now been reclassified as having PPMS. You might have been taking one or more DMTs, yet the disease continued to progress at a steady rate, without attacks and remissions. The diagnosis of PPMS is now made much more quickly, because of better understanding of the disease, improved awareness of this MS course, the development of magnetic resonance imaging (MRI), and better clinical criteria. Many people are now told that they probably have PPMS at the time of diagnosis or soon afterward.

I was diagnosed with PPMS right away. The neurologist based it on what I told him . . . I had no relapses, and I never got better.
— Jason

PPMS is characterized by a number of differences from the relapsing forms. Although no one individual will exhibit all of them, its most common features include:

► About 90 percent of people who are eventually diagnosed with PPMS begin by having difficulties with walking, in contrast to most people with RRMS, whose disease tends to begin with visual symptoms or numbness. At first, these problems might

We would walk around the lake, and about two-thirds of the way around my feet would start dragging. We just thought it was probably something like a pinched nerve. Four years went by before there was an actual diagnosis. — Kathy

be very subtle. People with PPMS notice that they have difficulty going up stairs and they tend to trip, especially when they are not concentrating on walking. Symptoms might be very mild for years before they talk to their doctor.

▶ Conversely, people with PPMS rarely exhibit visual difficulties or sensory problems such as numbness at the onset of the disease process.

▶ On MRI, people with PPMS have a smaller number of lesions and fewer gadolinium-enhancing lesions—which indicate active inflammation—than do people with RRMS. Not surprisingly, since walking is controlled by nerves originating in the spinal cord, people with PPMS tend to have more lesions in the spinal cord than in the brain. Having a substantial number of spinal cord lesions also means that bowel, bladder, and sexual function may be affected. On the positive side, this also means that people with PPMS often have less severe cognitive problems than do people with RRMS, although these may occur.

▶ Brain and spinal cord *atrophy*—an actual loss of mass of neural tissue—can be seen early in the course of PPMS, and this helps predict future disability. Atrophy appears as an increased volume in the *ventricles*—the fluid-filled cavities in the central region of the brain—and by a decrease in the diameter of the spinal cord on MRI.

▶ RRMS most commonly affects people in their 20s and 30s, whereas PPMS is commonly diagnosed later, often in the 40s or 50s. Because the average age at diagnosis for people with PPMS is about 10 years older than those with RRMS, the effects of age and age-related illness may complicate diagnosis. For example, the small brain lesions that occur with age can look very similar to MS on MRI.

▶ PPMS affects men and women equally, unlike RRMS, which affects women much more commonly, often reported as a ratio as high as 3:1. The reason for this is not clear, but women are more likely to develop a range of autoimmune diseases, which appears to include the inflammatory form of MS.

MAKING THE DIAGNOSIS OF PPMS

The basic characteristics of PPMS help neurologists make the diagnosis. Although a number of factors are common in PPMS, no single factor has been identified as a diagnostic marker. Instead, the diagnosis is based on clinical observation and examination, along with the pattern and combination of symptoms.

Guidelines for the Diagnosis of PPMS

A variety of criteria have been used to make the diagnosis of MS, beginning with the Schumacher criteria in 1965, which relied primarily on neurologic examination and the patient's history. Diagnosis became more straightforward with the advent of modern imaging techniques, as well as a variety of laboratory tests to measure immune reactions in the CNS. In 1983, the Poser criteria combined clinical findings with imaging and other test results.

I was a teacher of the deaf, and I was having trouble signing and finger spelling, and I couldn't understand what was happening. I had a five-year-old and a three-year-old, and I was running after them one day and couldn't run very fast. — Shelley

In 2001, the International Panel on the Diagnosis of Multiple Sclerosis proposed what became known as the *McDonald criteria*. One of its most important features was the use of MRI imaging to enhance the earlier reliance on clinical features for making a diagnosis. Although a diagnosis of MS could still be made on clinical observations alone—including multiple attacks and clear progression over time—MRI data indicating the kind, number, and location of demyelinating lesions indicative of MS allowed for earlier diagnosis in many cases.

These criteria were further refined in 2005, when the Panel made several changes of particular importance to people with PPMS, providing for increased consideration of spinal cord lesions and decreasing the emphasis on a positive cerebrospinal fluid (CSF) test in making a diagnosis of PPMS.

Despite these advances, identifying individuals with PPMS remains a challenge, especially early in the disease process. There is a strong need to tighten the definition of PPMS. This is not merely an academic issue; the lack of a definition and the ability to better characterize the processes involved in PPMS contribute to the lack of treatments.

Diagnosing RRMS requires evidence of at least two separate areas of damage in the CNS that have occurred at different points in time, with no other possible explanation. Although people with PPMS do experience a "waxing and waning," which might represent a form of "attack," they are not as dramatic as the attacks seen in RRMS.

2005 REVISED McDONALD DIAGNOSTIC CRITERIA FOR PPMS

▶ At least one year of progressively worsening neurologic symptoms suggestive of primary progressive multiple sclerosis, with no history of attacks or exacerbations.

AND

▶ Two out of three of the following:

- A "positive" brain MRI study PLUS positive results on visual evoked potential (VEP) testing indicating impaired transmissions in the optic nerve (behind the eye).

- A "positive" spinal cord MRI.

- A "positive" CSF test; meaning that the analysis of the fluid (obtained by lumbar puncture, often called a "spinal tap") indicates an abnormal immune response in the central nervous system that is consistent with MS.

Because they do not experience easily identifiable—or easily countable—inflammatory attacks, the diagnosis of PPMS requires somewhat different evidence:

The diagnostic process typically involves laboratory studies to rule out other diagnoses, MRI studies, CSF analysis, and evoked potentials studies. These tests are combined with the patient's history and physical examination.

Diagnosis remains difficult in the early stages of PPMS, and is often made only when a patient exhibits steady progression without relapses over a period of years. Clinicians and researchers are seeking markers of disease that will allow for an earlier diagnosis and the earlier initiation of management strategies. Although a number of factors have been identified as being more or less common in PPMS, to date no single factor has been identified that can serve as a diagnostic marker for this form of MS.

It is increasingly clear that the differences between PPMS and RRMS may be quantitative and not qualitative. Like the relapsing forms of MS, PPMS is believed to be an autoimmune disease, but the degree of inflammation is quantitatively less than that seen in the relapsing forms. It involves more atrophy and more disability.

Although this might suggest that individuals with PPMS should be treated with the same DMTs as people with RRMS, there is little evidence to suggest that DMTs are effective, and they are not approved by the Food and Drug Administration (FDA) for use in PPMS. There is some evidence that a different process may lead to inflammation in the two types. At present, some people with PPMS are on DMTs, reflecting the uncertainty about which patients are likely to respond.

When MRI came along, an MRI of my brain showed nothing, but they did find lesions on my spinal cord. Now I know that many men have spinal MS. That helped me realize that I'm not going to have exacerbations . . . instead I have a progressive disease.

— Tom

Several definable characteristics that predict progression include:

▶ Clinically, PPMS appears to be characterized by an early, steady progression.

▶ The distribution of lesions differs from that seen in RRMS and SPMS, with more spinal cord and fewer brain lesions.

▶ Brain and spinal cord atrophy can be seen early in the course of the disease, and these help to predict future disability. Atrophy is reflected by a general decrease in the amount of neural tissue and an increase in the amount of fluid that fills the spaces between neural tissue and the bony tissue of the cranium and spinal cord.

▶ The average age at diagnosis for people with PPMS is about 10 years later than for those with RRMS. Because they are older, they also tend to have other illnesses, often requiring more emphasis on differentiating other pathologic processes from MS.

Clinicians and researchers are aggressively seeking markers of disease that will allow for an earlier diagnosis and lead to improved therapeutic management.

What Tests Help to Make the Diagnosis of PPMS?

▶ **Magnetic resonance imaging (MRI):** This is the most sensitive noninvasive diagnostic tool used to view the brain and spinal cord and help establish the diagnosis of MS. It is also used to see how the disease is progressing after diagnosis. MRI uses a powerful magnetic field that produces detailed pictures of the tissue being examined. It clearly shows areas where myelin has been damaged. MS lesions appear as either a bright white spot or a darkened area, depending on the type of scan used.

▶ **Gadolinium (Gd) enhancement:** This substance can be injected intravenously during an MRI to further enhance the sensitivity of the scan and provide more accurate information about where damage has occurred and how extensive it is. A Gd-enhanced MRI scan supplies information about current disease activity by highlighting those areas of inflammation that represent new lesions, or ones that are becoming larger.

▶ **T1 and T2 lesions:** T1 images show "black holes," which are believed to indicate areas of permanent damage. T2-weighted MRI scans provide information about disease *burden* or *lesion load*—the total amount of lesion area.

▶ **Cerebrospinal fluid (CSF):** This clear, colorless liquid bathes the brain and spinal cord. It circulates nutrients and other substances filtered from the blood, removes waste products, and cushions these tissues by acting as a "shock absorber." The CSF of people with MS usually contains elevated levels of immunoglobulin G (IgG) antibodies and a group of proteins that appear as *oligoclonal bands*; it also contains the breakdown products of myelin. Samples of CSF are obtained through a lumbar puncture or "spinal tap."

▶ **Lumbar puncture (spinal tap):** In this procedure, a long, thin, hollow needle is inserted between two bones in the lower spine and into the space in which the CSF circulates. One to two tablespoonfuls of the fluid are then withdrawn for analysis.

▶ **Visual evoked potential (VEP):** VEP measures the electrical activity of the brain in response to stimulation of the visual pathway. It can help to confirm the diagnosis of MS by detecting the slowing of electrical conduction caused by demyelination along this pathway, even when the change is too subtle to be noticed by the person or show up on neurologic examination.

▶ **Expanded Disability Status Scale (EDSS):** This 20-point scale summarizes the neurologic examination and provides a measure of overall disability. It ranges by half-points from 0 (normal examination) to 10 (death due to MS).

▶ **MS Functional Composite (MSFC):** This three-part, standardized set of tests measures leg function/ambulation (Timed 25-Foot

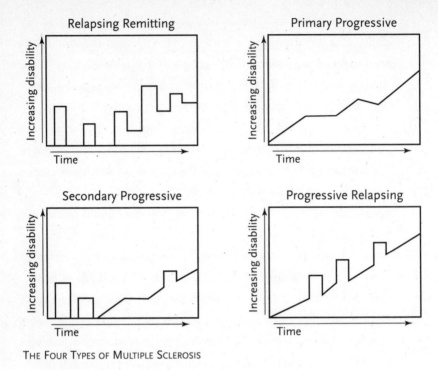

THE FOUR TYPES OF MULTIPLE SCLEROSIS

Walk), arm/hand function (Nine-Hole Peg Test), and cognitive function (Paced Auditory Serial Addition Test [PASAT]).

What Clinical Symptoms and Patterns Indicate the Diagnosis of PPMS?

The factors more commonly seen in PPMS are those that—in a reasonable combination—allow the diagnosis to be made:

► Major symptoms are related to difficulties with walking and mobility, as well as to other difficulties linked to lesions in the spinal cord, rather than problems such as visual symptoms or numbness.
► A history that involves steady progression without well-defined attacks and remissions is suggestive of PPMS.
► MRI findings that include relatively fewer brain lesions, especially Gd-enhancing lesions, are common in PPMS.

▶ The presence of brain and spinal cord atrophy is seen early in PPMS.

▶ When combined with one or more of the other indicators, an older age suggests the diagnosis of PPMS in people who have not experienced previous attacks or exacerbations.

▶ A man, especially one in his 40s or older, will often have PPMS rather than a relapsing-remitting form of MS.

How Do People with PPMS Differ from Those with SPMS?

The word "progressive" is also associated with the form of MS that occurs in people whose disease began as RRMS. With time, their pattern of disease—defined as SPMS—changes from one that involves relapses and remissions to one characterized by steady progression with fewer or no attacks. Although significant clinical similarities exist between SPMS and RRMS, there are also significant differences between them.

I suggested to my neurologist that I thought it was primary progressive MS, because the symptoms were just constantly getting worse. When I finally saw a neurologist who specialized in MS, he sent me in to have a spinal MRI . . . I'd only had brain MRIs. When he looked at those, there were quite a few very classic lesions on the spine. — Kathy

As noted earlier, people with PPMS do not experience attacks and remissions; individuals with SPMS may have a limited number of attacks superimposed on an increasingly steady progression.

The distribution of lesions is different in the two forms. People with PPMS have more lesions around the ventricles than do those with RRMS that has progressed to SPMS. People with PPMS also have more lesions in the cervical (neck) region of the spinal cord. This difference might explain why people with PPMS have more symptoms associated with damage to the spinal cord.

2

How Is Primary Progressive Multiple Sclerosis Managed?

What do we mean when we discuss *managing* primary progressive multiple sclerosis (PPMS)? In its broadest sense, management encompasses a wide range of strategies, including controlling the actual disease process, managing its symptoms, encouraging overall wellness, managing emotional and family issues, and dealing with the economic issues that result from living with a chronic disease. Many options and strategies can help you achieve and maintain optimal functioning and wellness in the presence of PPMS. These options are discussed in detail in the chapters that follow. Your team of health care professionals will help determine the best approaches for *you.*

MODIFYING THE PPMS DISEASE COURSE: AN ELUSIVE GOAL

Unlike relapsing remitting MS (RRMS), no treatment to date has shown convincing evidence of slowing the accumulation of disability for people with PPMS, and no medications are approved by the Food and Drug Administration (FDA) for its treatment. The *good* news is that new treatments are in clinical trials. Recently completed clinical trials provide some hope that researchers are on a favorable track for future treatments.

The reasons for this are discussed in detail in Chapter 3. Despite evidence indicating that the disease modifying therapies (DMTs) used in RRMS do not appear to be effective in PPMS, the data are not yet conclusive, and at the time of this writing many people with PPMS are on one of these therapies.

WHY AM I RECEIVING A DISEASE MODIFYING THERAPY IF I HAVE PPMS?

The role of inflammation in PPMS is not well understood, but it probably differs from that in RRMS. Some people with PPMS have fluctuating symptoms that resemble relapsing MS, and early symptoms may overlap with those seen in relapsing MS. Each person's disease course is unique, and at first you might not fit precisely within one pattern or another. Additionally, some people with PPMS experience a sense that their disease progression is lessened on their current therapies. For these reasons, a doctor might decide to use one of the currently approved therapies for relapsing MS until the disease course is more clearly defined.

The currently approved DMTs include the interferon beta medications (Avonex®, Betaseron®, Rebif®, and the recently approved Extavia®) and Copaxone®. All are approved by the FDA for use in the *relapsing forms* of MS, and these agents work primarily by reducing immune system activity as indicated by a demonstrated clinical slowing of progression and a reduced number of acute relapses and number of new lesions on MRI scans. If they are not effective or their side effects are not tolerable, a physician might recommend changing to another therapy in this group or trying Tysabri® (natalizumab) or Novantrone® (mitoxantrone) in relapsing forms of MS.

Prescribing a medication for something other than its approved use is known as "prescribing off-label." However, many insurance companies are unwilling to pay for an off-label use of a medication, especially the expensive DMTs used in MS. If a doctor believes that the medication is appropriate for a particular reason, even though it has not been approved for use in PPMS, he or she can appeal the company's decision.

A great deal can be done to manage PPMS, even for people who are not considered good candidates for a DMT. These topics are discussed in detail in later chapters on symptom management, rehabilitation, overall health and wellness, social support systems, and emotional well-being—all of which have important benefits for everyone with PPMS and their families.

As with other chronic illnesses and disorders, PPMS is best managed by a comprehensive approach that moves away from the "medical" model of care toward a "functional" model in which the concerns of patients, family members, and caregivers play a key role, with services provided by a wide variety of knowledgeable health care professionals to meet your specific needs. A comprehensive approach to management may include the following strategies:

> *No doctor really looked me in the eyes and told me there is no cure and there is no treatment. It took me about 2 years to realize that myself.*
> *— Jason*

▶ **Rehabilitation to maximize function:** The members of the PPMS "team" are discussed in detail in Chapter 4. While we await treatments to prevent damage or restore central nervous system (CNS) function, the broad group of management strategies that are encompassed by the term *rehabilitation* can be used to help you take advantage of the many strengths that you might not be aware you have.

▶ **Symptom management:** Symptom management is essential to maintaining comfort and productivity, as well as to enhancing quality of life. Chapter 5 reviews the many therapies that can alleviate symptoms and improve your physical function.

▶ **Enhancing mobility and promoting safety and independence:** Chapter 6 discusses the wide range of technologies and adaptations to your home, environment, and work environment that can make your life easier and enhance your independence both at home and in the community.

▶ **Promoting overall health and wellness:** Maintaining optimal health in the presence of PPMS can be a challenge. Chapter 7 discusses a wide range of strategies that are available to assure that your overall quality of life is good. The role of exercise and good nutrition is emphasized, as well as the many wellness strategies that can make a difference, such as managing stress.

▶ **Coping with emotional issues:** Many people tend to neglect their emotional health because they are focused on managing physical symptoms. However, managing emotional issues can go a long way toward maintaining a good quality of life. Chapter 8 provides basic strategies for dealing with these problems.

▶ **Family issues:** PPMS affects all areas of family life, including relationships with spouses and children, as well as the family's relationships within the community. Chapter 9 discusses strategies for coping effectively, including the development of a *carepartnership*, intimacy issues, parenting, and much more. Chapter 10 focuses on home care and related issues for advanced PPMS.

▶ **Economic issues:** Living with a chronic disease such as PPMS can present many problems of an economic nature, including employment concerns, financial planning, and insurance issues. These are discussed in Chapter 11.

The goal of these strategies is to increase *quality of life*, a feeling that can be achieved by enhancing relationships, productivity, and creativity. A final chapter on *How the Multiple Sclerosis Organizations Can Help* discusses a wide range of services that can help you in all areas of living with PPMS. In addition, the appendices include a glossary of common terms and an extensive resource section, which makes this book an excellent "jumping off" place in managing PPMS.

There wasn't much Shelley didn't try, including having her fillings removed.
— Dave

Research and Clinical Trials

Research studying any disease has two components: basic and clinical. Basic research is the first step of many before a new therapy can be tested in people. It often begins in a sterile laboratory and involves exploring how cells function outside the body, or *in vitro*. This is followed by a series of human clinical trials. All of this must occur before any new treatment becomes available for general use, and most potential therapies fail somewhere along the way. Success usually takes many years at a cost that can reach several hundred million dollars.

People are often frustrated by the relatively small number of clinical trials in primary progressive multiple sclerosis (PPMS) compared to those ongoing for relapsing remitting MS (RRMS). Fewer clinical trials focus on PPMS for several important reasons:

▶ We have less understanding of the process underlying PPMS than we do of other types of MS. Unless the mechanism by which a disease occurs is understood, it is difficult to develop a drug that will directly affect the disease process.

▶ PPMS can be more difficult to diagnose or to distinguish from other disease courses, at least initially.

▶ The slowly progressing course of the disease makes it more difficult to see an immediate effect of a new drug.

▶ There are no easily identifiable outcome measures to use in clinical trials, such as the number of relapses and the number of new lesions seen on MRI over the course of a two- or three-year trial—the most common measures used to study relapsing MS.

▶ Because PPMS is the least common MS course, it is difficult to recruit the number of people needed to participate in a clinical trial in order to analyze the results in a meaningful way.

▶ No good animal model of PPMS exists that is analogous to experimental autoimmune encephalomyelitis (EAE) for RRMS. In RRMS, a significant amount of preclinical basic scientific research has already been done for therapies designed to treat this form of MS.

▶ Currently available disease modifying therapies (DMTs) act by controlling inflammation, a major characteristic of relapsing MS. These medications do not seem to be as effective in PPMS.

When people with PPMS *are* included in clinical trials, it tends to be for agents developed to manage symptoms. Fortunately, this is a crucial issue for people with PPMS, because better symptom management translates into better overall health and quality of life.

The best news is that new research in areas that have the potential to affect the PPMS disease process is leading to new and exciting information that offers the hope of future management therapies. New drug trials are now aimed at helping people with PPMS.

THE IMMUNE SYSTEM IN MULTIPLE SCLEROSIS

Understanding the basics of how the immune system works is important. Research on MS has focused intensively on this system, and the DMTs used for RRMS (and sometimes for PPMS) are aimed at modifying immune function.

The immune system is the body's defense against viruses, bacteria, toxins, and other substances from outside the body, as well as against

How Do the Relapsing and Progressive Forms of MS Differ?

Until recently, damage in the relapsing forms of MS was thought to be related to inflammation only, while the damage in PPMS was thought to be caused by a degenerative process. These concepts are now being challenged. The relapsing forms of MS have now been shown to involve a degenerative process as well as inflammation; conversely, the damage in PPMS appears to have an immunologic component along with degeneration.

People with PPMS often experience a "waxing and waning," with periods during which the disease seems to be worse alternating with periods when it is relatively better. These periods are less distinct than those seen in relapsing MS and cannot necessarily be identified objectively by examination—that is, they do not appear to have identifiable or quantifiable features that can be measured in the neurologic examination.

abnormal cells such as those that cause cancer. Cells of the immune system react against "nonself" substances that don't belong in the body. For example, immune cells initiate the inflammation that occurs at the site of a cut or insect bite and the reaction against viruses when you have the flu.

The immune system includes the skin as the first-line barrier to outside organisms; lymph, bone, marrow, thymus, and other organs; a variety of white blood cell types; and the products of those cells, including antibodies that target invading agents such as viruses and bacteria.

An *autoimmune* disease occurs when the body's immune system reacts against a substance normally recognized as "self," causing it to attack its own tissues. Most researchers believe that MS involves an autoimmune process. The molecule that is attacked is thought to be a component of *myelin*, which, as previously discussed, provides protection and insulation for the wiring (axons) and neurons in the central nervous system (CNS). Myelin is required for normal transmission of the electrical impulses throughout the nervous system to control muscles, as well as for internal communications within the brain and spinal cord. One theory is that a genetically susceptible person's immune system reacts to a variety of viral or other infections and environmental exposure in childhood, and is somehow "set up" to have her or his immune system later attack the CNS. Although many potential triggers have been studied, including viruses (such as Epstein-Barr virus, which casues mononucleosis) and bacteria, we have still not identified the "cause" of MS. Other environmental factors are likely to play a role; for example, some research suggests that vitamin D might be involved in a complex interaction with genetic makeup.

I don't think we could even remember all the things we tried. I did megadoses of steroids, ACTH, intravenous methyl-prednisolone, an NIH study with plasmapheresis, chemotherapy. I even tried hyperbaric oxygen and bee stings. — Shelley

Most studies of MS focus on the two major white blood cell types involved in autoimmune reactions, T and B cells, both of which are *lymphocytes*. Receptors on T cells have the ability to recognize specific molecules, called *antigens*, such as proteins from infecting organisms. Once the antigen is identified, specific T cells, called *helper T cells*, trigger the B cells to release *antibodies* or *immunoglobulins*. These are Y-shaped proteins that bind to specific antigens. These proteins fit into the molecular structure of the invading substance in a way that is often referred to as a "lock-and-key" mechanism. After the lymphocytes respond to an antigen, they signal other white blood cells to gather at the injured or infected site to destroy the invading factors or antigens through a process that involves *inflammation*.

Cells of the immune system also produce substances called *cytokines*, some of which stimulate the immune reaction, while others decrease it. In addition, many cells produce *interferons*; several of the drugs used to reduce inflammation in the relapsing forms of MS are beta interferons. However, some other interferons (gamma interferons) can increase inflammation.

Most MS research has focused on T cells, because the relapsing forms of the disease appear to be related to a misdirection of the T-cells, and most of the presently approved drugs for treating MS appear to primarily affect T cells. If the damage in PPMS is related to immune system factors other than T cells (such as antibodies), the lack of advances in managing PPMS becomes easier to understand. Many researchers are now addressing this problem.

CLINICAL TRIALS

How Are Clinical Trials Conducted?

Clinical trials are an essential step before a promising new drug or other medical therapy can be evaluated by the U.S. Food and Drug Administration (FDA) for safety and effectiveness. The National Institutes of Health (NIH), the National MS Society, or pharmaceutical and biotechnology companies sponsor clinical trials in MS (for more information, see: www.nationalmssociety.org/research/clinical-trials/clinical-trial-resources/index.aspx, or www.clinicaltrials.gov).

Trials are usually conducted in steps, called *phases*, and these almost always follow substantial laboratory research. By the time human testing begins, the manufacturer is confident that the drug stands a good chance of meeting the need for which it was developed and that it will likely be safe. In some cases, drugs undergoing testing in the U.S. have already been approved in Europe or elsewhere. Depending on the quality and nature of these studies, these data may shorten the trial in the U.S.

▶ Phase I trials usually enroll a small number of people (20–80), last about a year, and determine whether the drug is safe and the study should be continued. They evaluate what dose is safe, how a new agent should be given, how often it should be given, and whether it has any harmful side effects.

▶ Phase II trials often involve 100–300 people and can last several years. Participants are usually divided into a group that receives the active drug and a *control group* that receives either an existing treatment or a *placebo.*

▶ Phase III trials are the last step before a drug is approved by the FDA for general use. They can involve 1,000–3,000 people and can last for up to 5 years. To be approved, a new drug must be at least as effective as one or more treatments already in use, and/or be demonstrably better than a placebo.

▶ Phase IV trials further evaluate the long-term safety and effectiveness of a treatment after it is approved. Additional uses can also be explored. Several hundred to several thousand people might take part in the trial, and any problems must be reported to the FDA.

Many years can elapse between early laboratory research and an approved treatment, and the time and effort involved come at an enormous cost. Most potential treatments fail because they are ineffective or toxic.

How Are Clinical Trials Designed?

The best clinical trials are prospective, randomized, cross-over, and double-blinded studies. You will see these terms frequently in any discussion of clinical trials.

▶ **Prospective:** Participants are identified before the study begins and then followed-up with over time.

▶ **Randomized:** Participants are grouped by chance, usually through a computer program. One group receives the treatment being evaluated and the other receives either the current standard treatment or a placebo.

▶ **Cross-over:** Each participant receives both the treatment and a placebo, but at different times.

▶ **Double-blinded:** Neither the participants nor the researchers know which group a participant is in.

▶ **Open label:** Both the participants and the treating researchers know that the participant is receiving the treatment and not a placebo. However, the evaluating physician researcher is usually not aware of the specific treatment given to the patient.

Eligibility Criteria

Every clinical trial has guidelines, called *eligibility criteria*, about who can or cannot participate in the study. They describe characteristics that must be shared by all participants—these might include age, gender, previous treatment history, and other medical conditions—and they often require that participants have a particular type and stage of MS. Enrolling individuals with similar characteristics helps ensure that researchers will be able to achieve accurate and meaningful results.

For information on how to learn more about ongoing clinical trials in PPMS, see Appendix 2.

Completed Clinical Trials

Several recent trials have failed to meet their endpoints of clearly demonstrating an effect on slowing the progression of PPMS, but their results suggest directions that might be useful in future studies.

▶ **The PROMISe trial** of Copaxone® (glatiramer acetate) in 943 people with PPMS was stopped early because it failed to reach its effectiveness endpoint. However, a post-study analysis suggested that the drug might have been effective in the 14 percent of participants who had gadolinium (Gd)-enhancing lesions, which is indicative of active inflammation. Some of the male participants might have had some benefit.

▶ **Studies of interferons beta-1a and beta-1b, and mitoxantrone** generally failed to meet their clinical or magnetic resonance imaging (MRI) effectiveness endpoints, which included reductions in time to sustained disability, lesion load, and atrophy of the brain and spinal cord. However, there was a trend toward a slower progression rate in several of these studies, and future studies will attempt to obtain more conclusive data.

▶ **The OLYMPUS trial** in 439 individuals of Rituxan® (rituximab), a monoclonal antibody that inhibits the activity of B cells (to produce antibodies), failed to achieve its primary endpoint. However, a post-study analysis showed that individuals under age 55 with Gd-enhancing (Gd+) lesions, which is indicative of inflammation, might have responded to the drug. Older individuals who had the disease for many years did not appear to respond.

These studies suggest that, with careful participant selection, it might be possible to achieve measurable improvement in at least some individuals with PPMS. However, none of the potential beneficiary effects in studies to date are robust enough to allow FDA approval, and more studies are needed.

POTENTIALLY RELEVANT NEW RESEARCH

At this time, most FDA-approved DMTs for relapsing MS focus on T cells. However, newer potential PPMS therapies are targeting those B cells that control the antibody part of the immune system. Other new strategies are aimed at protecting axons and myelin from being damaged (neuroprotection) or at restoring lost function (remyelination).

An example of a new potential PPMS treatment illustrates some of the results of new research to help people with PPMS. The Phase III INFORMS study of fingolimod (FTY720) for people with PPMS began in early 2009, and participants were being recruited as this book was in development. This study will evaluate whether the drug delays the progression of disability compared to a placebo in patients treated for at least 36 months. Secondary outcome measures include evaluation of safety and tolerability, as well as the effect of the drug on MRI and patient-reported outcomes. The estimated enrollment is 654 individuals, and the estimated completion date is 2013.

Participants must be between the ages of 25 and 65, have a diagnosis of PPMS, have first reported symptoms within the previous 2–10 years, show evidence of disease progression within the previous 2 years, and have an Expanded Disability Status Scale (EDSS; disability rating) of 3.5–6.0. No one will be enrolled who has a history of relapses or certain other medical conditions.

Ongoing Research on PPMS

Current research is focused on determining whether specific subgroups of people with PPMS might be amenable to treatment. It might be possible to identify people with PPMS who are more likely to respond to therapy based on characteristics that can be identified by clinical patterns or tests such as MRI or cerebrospinal fluid (CSF) analysis. Might early PPMS be more easily treated? Might PPMS with inflammation or lesions on MRI (Gd-enhancing lesions) respond better? Are other factors present that might favor specific treatments? For example, in the PROMISe trial discussed earlier, evidence suggested that the drug may have helped men more than women. Participants with lesions on MRI appeared more likely to progress than those who did not, as did participants with a higher overall *burden of disease* as defined by the number and size of lesions on MRI.

Nervous System Repair, Protection, and Regeneration

Researchers are studying possible mechanisms that might prevent new damage to brain tissue and restore function in people who have already experienced significant nervous system damage. People with PPMS will be candidates for future CNS repair and protection strategies. (For a detailed overview of research in MS, visit the National MS Society's website www.nationalmssociety.org, and download the file *Research Directions in Multiple Sclerosis*.)

One of the most exciting areas of current research is to develop ways to promote repair of the damaged tissue in MS, possibly by inducing the body's own cells to more adequately carry out the repair function or by introducing replacement cells from a different source. Recent scientific advances in many different fields are now coming together to bring the dream of protecting and repairing brain tissue, and restoring function within our grasp. This research has the potential to show us how to stop disease progression, thereby improving the quality of life for people living with MS.

Several strategies to stimulate myelin repair are now ongoing:

▶ Researchers are trying to identify the molecular signals used by the body to activate young *oligodendrocytes*—myelin-producing cells—so that those signals can be mimicked in a controlled fashion to stimulate additional repair.

▶ A large group of proteins—known as "growth factors" for their roles in "turning on" different stages of myelin formation and nerve growth—are the focus of extensive research.

▶ Another approach is to identify and block natural processes that might inhibit the body's ability to repair nervous system damage.

▶ Scientists are working to identify potential sources of replacement cells for those damaged by MS; this takes us into the field of stem cell research. The usefulness of these possible replacement cells will depend on many factors, including finding or creating the signals needed to stimulate their transformation and growth into healthy new cells. Many challenges await these efforts.

Maintaining Axonal Structure and Function

As previously discussed, axons conduct electrical brain impulses, or messages. They are insulated by myelin. Myelin appears to help maintain axon structure and function, and axonal breakdown seems to be a consequence of demyelination. The extent of axonal breakdown in animal models may help us better understand the mechanisms by which this breakdown occurs. New research is focused on using nerve cell cultures exposed to destructive substances in the presence or absence of other substances that are either potentially protective or that provide growth signals to stimulate repair and/or growth of new cells. The results of these laboratory experiments could potentially be used to develop new PPMS treatments in clinical trials.

Myelin Protection

A protein in myelin called MAG (myelin-associated glycoprotein) is found in the brain and spinal cord. Under certain conditions, it can either stop or promote axonal growth, and its presence could block the migration of myelin-making cells to repair the damaged areas. Understanding how this myelin protein works could lead to new ways to protect or repair nerves in MS.

Proteins released by immune T cells not only damage nerve cells, they inhibit the cells that are trying to repair the brain. By understanding which proteins are the most important, we may be able to reduce inflammation and allow natural reparative processes to occur more efficiently.

Future research studies will include pilot trials of neuroprotective and neuroregeneration strategies in people with MS, based on information gained from this type of research.

Repairing Nervous System Damage in Laboratory Studies

Possible ways of repairing nervous system damage are being studied in rodents (usually mice), utilizing the MS-like disease EAE. In this model, immature myelin-making cells from the brain are transplanted into animals, and their ability to form myelin is studied.

Studies are also ongoing to find out whether remyelination can be enhanced using transplants of cells involved in this process. This is based on the discovery that neural stem cells will enter the brain from the bloodstream and enhance remyelination in mice.

Neuroprotective Agents

Numerous drugs have been found to protect the nervous system from damage. They are now being tested in EAE, both as individual compounds or in combinations.

Although the body has some nerve-tissue repair capabilities, these eventually fail in MS—possibly because the body's store of immature myelin-making cells is depleted or because there is a lack of growth factors to stimulate tissue repair. These possibilities are now being studied using the EAE model.

Prospects for Cell Therapy and Stem Cell Research

Stem cell research is not new. Stem cells retain the ability to renew themselves through cell division, and they can differentiate and develop into a diverse range of specialized cell types. They have been used for years in bone marrow transplantation. The human body appears to offer an almost limitless source of replacement cells.

Animal studies are now being done to work out safety issues relating to the use of new cells to repair MS-related damage, to find the optimal source of cells to transplant, to determine how to obtain enough cells for transplant, and to find the best mode of delivery. Some might be used to treat MS if the appropriate signals that stimulate remyelination can be identified, and if safe, effective therapeutic agents are developed that will stimulate this process.

How Does Rehabilitation Maintain and Improve Function?

A diagnosis of primary progressive multiple sclerosis (PPMS) brings many questions about what the future will hold, both medically and in terms of your personal life: Will I need to use a wheelchair? What about my job? How will the disease affect my thinking? Will I be less able to be a good spouse and parent? What about insurance?

> Rehabilitation encompasses a wide variety of strategies and therapies designed to help you reach and then maintain the best physical, emotional, and functional level possible, whatever your level of disability. It will help improve function to the maximum extent possible by managing symptoms, promoting independence regardless of the severity of PPMS, and help you maintain a high quality of life (QOL). A rehabilitation program should be individually designed to deal with specific symptoms, problems, and life circumstances.

No one can answer these questions with any certainty, because PPMS varies widely from person to person, and there is no "typical" pattern of progression or development of disability. Some people experience periods during which their progression seems to level off, while others become disabled more quickly. At times, you may feel that you can no longer trust your body, and your previous expectations of good heath will be turned upside down. It is important to remember that people and resources are available every step of the way to help with whatever the future brings.

Even without an approved disease modifying therapy (DMT), people with PPMS and their health care teams can do a great deal to manage the disease, including:

▶ Managing symptoms
▶ Enhancing mobility and promoting safety and independence
▶ Promoting overall health and wellness
▶ Promoting emotional well-being and quality of life
▶ Preventing complications, such as bladder infections

A key concept in rehabilitation has traditionally been the distinction among the terms *impairment, disability,* and *handicap.* Impairment refers to any loss or abnormality of function as experienced by the body. A disability is a substantial limitation in function as experienced by the affected individual, and a handicap is the resulting social limitations that affect the interactions between the individual and his environment. An example as it might occur in MS relates to spasticity. The impairment is the condition of spasticity; the disability is the inability to use the affected limb properly; and the handicap is the effect on the ability to navigate in the home and community. Although you may continue to see these terms for some time, the new World Health Organization's (WHO) International Classification of Function refers instead to "health condition, body structure, and function," and the consideration of how these

"When you have lemons, how do you make lemonade?" That's probably a good theme for anyone with MS. You'd never wish to have it, but since you do, and since you have some limitations, how do you continue to function and do those things that you want to do that you find rewarding in spite of it? — Kathy

and "environmental and personal factors" affect a person's level of "activity and participation" in the community. Over the next few years, these terms will come to replace the older ones because they are more appropriate in terms of an individual's life.

Focusing on rehabilitation will help you relearn skills or find new ways of doing things that have become difficult. It often involves physical therapy (PT) to help your strength, mobility, and fitness; occupational therapy (OT) to help with your daily activities; speech-language therapy to help with speaking, understanding, reading, writing, and swallowing; and specialists in pain management.

The goals of rehabilitation include:

▶ Helping you reach the highest possible level of function and comfort possible, given the limitations that result from PPMS
▶ Helping you maintain that level of function as long as possible
▶ Preventing unnecessary and potentially dangerous complications
▶ Providing you with any assistive devices you need to conserve energy and carry out your daily activities effectively, safely, and comfortably

Optimally, rehabilitation is provided by a team of specialists, with *you* as its center (Figure 4.1). At a comprehensive MS center or clinic, many or most of these team members will be affiliated with the center. Neurologists or other specialist physicians who practice independently or with a group of specialists will create the team through referrals.

The rehabilitation team includes, but is not limited to, the following specialists:

▶ **Neurologists** normally diagnose MS and PPMS, prescribe and manage DMTs, and manage PPMS symptoms. Your neurologist must be seen on a regular basis—usually several times a year. He or she will evaluate your MS, review your medications, recommend any new management strategies that might be helpful, and make referrals to other medical specialists when necessary.

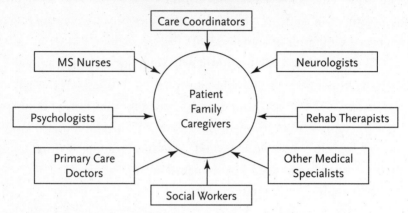

Integrated Medical and Functional Model
Patient Centered and Seamless

FIGURE 4.1   THE REHABILITATION TEAM

▶ **Other physicians** will treat issues associated with PPMS, as well as all general medical and surgical care that might or might not be related to MS. Your internist, family practitioner, or other general medical specialist will continue to oversee general medical care and regular screening tests—such as colonoscopies and mammograms—designed to detect other diseases at the earliest possible time.

▶ **Nurses, nurse practitioners (NPs), and physicians assistants (PAs)** are often the "managers" who coordinate overall care and wellness-related issues. A primary goal of nursing care in PPMS is to help with learning effective, preventive self-care, in order to manage minor problems before they become major ones. Some nurses and PAs provide follow-up care and help coordinate clinical trials.

▶ **Physical therapists (PTs)** treat problems that involve mobility and ambulation, balance, coordination, strength, pain, and fatigue.

I have people come several times a week, and they move my legs and arms so that I can keep mobile and not freeze in a certain position. I also have a standing frame, where I can stand up and practice getting upright.

That feels really good, to be off my bottom. — Shelley

The goal of physical therapy is to help manage the mobility challenges and physical demands of your family, work, and social life that are caused by PPMS. A PT can suggest an appropriate exercise program, and should be consulted regarding the proper use of rehabilitation equipment and mobility devices.

▶ **Occupational therapists** (OTs) can help you maintain the everyday skills you need to function as independently as possible. They focus on four major areas:

- Upper body strength, movement, and coordination
- Aids to independent living, such as the use of technology and environmental modifications
- Compensatory strategies for symptoms, including sensation problems, weakness, or vision loss
- Energy conservation

OTs will also be able to assist you with activities such as dressing, bathing, grooming, meal preparation, and writing, as well as managing a job, going to school, driving, and participating in leisure activities.

▶ **Speech and language pathologists** evaluate and treat problems that might result from damage to the nerves controlling muscles used in speech and swallowing. They also evaluate and treat communication issues related to cognitive deficits, such as problems with attention, memory, finding the words to express ideas while speaking or writing, and processing or remembering what is heard or read.

▶ **Mental health professionals** include psychiatrists, psychologists, and neuropsychologists, and licensed professional counselors such as social workers. They can help you deal with the many emotional issues that can affect your overall ability to adjust to living with PPMS.

▶ **Social workers** also can help you deal with any changes and adjustments that need to be made in coping with PPMS on a daily basis. They can assess social and family needs, and refer you to community service organizations that can assist you with income

maintenance, insurance, housing, long-term care options, counseling, and many other issues.

▶ **Other team members** might include vocational rehabilitation specialists; recreational therapists; spiritual counselors such as minis-
ters, priests, and rabbis; attorneys for legal assistance; nutritionists;
and many others.

Subsequent chapters discuss how you and your family can better
manage living with PPMS, and you will learn more about these specialists and the ways they can be helpful.

5

Symptom Management: Treatment Options

Primary progressive multiple sclerosis (PPMS) can produce a wide range of symptoms, in a variety of combinations. We usually consider symptoms to fall into three categories: primary, secondary, or tertiary.

Primary symptoms directly result from the disease process. They include fatigue, weakness, spasticity, tremor, poor coordination, and other problems that affect mobility, bladder and bowel issues, sexual difficulties, pain, dizziness and visual problems, speech and swallowing difficulties, and cognitive impairment.

Secondary symptoms do not directly result from the disease process, but are a consequence of primary symptoms. For example, contractures (frozen joints) can result from advanced spasticity, falls and other injuries can result from not using appropriate assistive devices to manage walking difficulties, malnutrition can result from swallowing disorders, and pressure sores can result from immobility. These complications can be prevented by good management, as discussed below and in Chapter 4.

Tertiary symptoms include the psychological, social, and economic issues that may result from living with PPMS, such as financial and employment concerns, role changes within the family, and decreased independence. Assistance with these types of issues can be provided by psychologists, social workers, counselors, and other professionals.

Because PPMS is primarily a spinal cord disease, the symptoms that cause the most difficulty are the result of damage to this area. These include spasticity and lower extremity weakness; bowel and bladder problems, including urinary tract infections; sexual difficulties; and issues related to skin care resulting from lack of mobility.

Because disability is common with PPMS, symptom management and the support systems that help people deal with them must be aggressive. This chapter discusses the optimal management of primary symptoms and the prevention of secondary ones, while later chapters deal with emotional, psychosocial, and interpersonal issues.

For a more detailed discussion of symptom management, we refer you to several sources, including the individual symptoms listed on the National MS Society's website at www.nationalmssociety.org; the article *MS Symptom Management Update 2009* by Diana M. Schneider, Ph.D., which can be downloaded from the MS Association of America's website at www.msassociation.org/publications/winter09/cover.story.asp; and the book *Managing the Symptoms of Multiple Sclerosis* by Randall T. Schapiro, M.D.

> Prescribing a medication for something other than its approved use is known as "prescribing off-label." In other words, the physician is prescribing the medication for a purpose other than the use(s) listed in its U.S. Food and Drug Administration (FDA)-approved labeling. This is not uncommon, and many of the medications used to treat MS symptoms are prescribed off-label because they have never been approved specifically for use in MS.

FATIGUE

We begin with fatigue because it is one of the most disabling symptoms for many people with PPMS. Another term sometimes used is "lassitude," an overwhelming sense of tiredness, lack of energy, or feeling of exhaustion. This type of fatigue usually comes without warning and is not related to exertion. It can be chronic, severe, or on-and-off, and it can occur at any stage of PPMS. When present, it affects everything else—from walking to cognition—and you will see repeated references to the effect of fatigue on other symptoms throughout this chapter.

> It's always a matter of cost/benefit. How much is this worth? If I do this, maybe I won't be able to go out tonight. Everything is like that, absolutely everything.
> — Shelley

Fatigue can also result from sleep deprivation, depression and anxiety, and a variety of medications—including those used to treat both the other symptoms of MS and non–MS-related conditions. It is important that your health provider address these problems with a comprehensive checkup if you are experiencing fatigue.

Once these factors have been ruled out or treated, fatigue can frequently be relieved by energy-conserving approaches, such as scheduling rest periods during the day, increasing your fitness level through exercise and good nutrition, and cooling techniques. Stress management techniques and meditation can also be helpful.

Because many people with MS are heat-sensitive and find that their fatigue is increased in hot weather or in warm indoor environments, a variety of cooling techniques have been found to be useful. These include swimming in cool water, taking cool drinks on warm days, using air conditioning, and using a cooling vest.

You might see a pattern to your fatigue; for example, many people experience it most in the afternoon. An occupational therapist (OT) can help you plan your activities to take advantage of those times when you tend to have the most energy, and to pace your activities to allow for rest periods, so you are able to enjoy the things you most want to do.

A number of drugs are effective in managing fatigue. Many were developed to treat other disorders, such as decreased alertness or depression. They include Provigil® (modafinil), which promotes wakefulness; amantadine, originally developed as an antiviral medication used to prevent or treat influenza; Ritalin® (methylphenidate), originally developed as a treatment for attention deficit disorder and also used to manage narcolepsy; Dexedrine® (dextroamphetamine), a stimulant that may improve wakefulness, boost energy, and decrease fatigue and appetite; a variety of antidepressant medications; and caffeine, taken as coffee, tea, or caffeinated soda.

SYMPTOMS THAT AFFECT MOBILITY

Because people with PPMS tend to have more spinal cord lesions than those with other forms of MS, the onset of PPMS is most often characterized by gradually increasing problems with walking. Lesions in the spinal cord can also cause bladder and bowel symptoms, as well as sexual dysfunction and fatigue. Lesions in the brain could cause other symptoms to develop, including visual disturbance, cognitive problems, mood changes, balance problems, and tremor, among others. However, there is no way to predict this, and your primary challenge may continue to be walking.

Every time I want to do something like take off a sweater or a jacket or put something on, I have to figure out how I'm going to do it and how much energy I'll have to spend doing it. Sometimes I just don't do things because I don't want to waste the energy. Sometimes, I'll sit in my wheelchair because I don't want to take the effort to get out of it.
— Shelley

Spasticity

Spasticity is characterized by an increase in muscle tone that causes stiffness and pain. It is especially common in the legs, and can be one of the most disturbing symptoms in PPMS. When mild, it may make it difficult to walk or limit the distance that can be walked. If not treated properly, severe spasticity can result in contractures—an inability to fully straighten a joint—that can permanently bend and limit movement of the joints at the arms, legs, or

shoulders, and which may also contribute to the development of pressure sores, as well as to abnormal posture and falls. A physical therapist
(PT) can help you avoid these problems, espe-
cially by providing strategies to minimize potentially dangerous falls.

The first step in managing spasticity is to
check for other conditions that may be causing
the problem, including other PPMS symptoms
as well as non–PPMS-related issues. These might
include fatigue, stress, heat, urinary tract and
other infections, and pain. Therapies designed to
relieve these symptoms may significantly
improve spasticity.

After other medical causes are ruled out,
spasticity can be reduced by regular stretching,
proper positioning in bed (side-lying with supports for the back and legs), range-of-motion
(ROM) exercises, and physical therapy. A PT can
develop a stretching program for your specific
needs; aquatic exercise might also be helpful.

*I sit in front of the
computer all day and
produce movies. The
physical therapist
really stretches me
out, because my
muscles get a lot
tighter with sitting.
I do calisthenics, and
then endurance and
strength exercises. I
do like upper body
cardio, because I
can't do it with my
lower body. When I
don't do physical
therapy, I tighten up.
— Jason*

Baclofen is the most commonly used med-
ication to manage spasticity; it works to reduce muscle stiffness and the
frequency and intensity of spasms. It can also be delivered directly into the
spinal fluid through a small catheter threaded into the spinal canal,
directed by a computerized pump programmed to deliver the appropriate
dose. This involves a minor surgical procedure that is generally straightforward. Other medications include Zanaflex® (tizanidine), Valium®
(diazepam), Klonopin® (clonazepam), and Neurontin® (gabapentin).
Fampridine SR® (4-aminopyridine) which improves impulse conduction
in demyelinated nerve fibers, may be helpful in some individuals.

If these medications do not provide adequate relief, it is possible
to inject either Botox® or Myobloc® (botulinum toxin) into affected
muscles to allow them to relax. This is usually used for *localized* spas-

I have always had some sort of range-of-motion exercises. I'm very disabled. My legs don't work very well. My right arm is somewhat useful, but not all of it, because my dexterity is not great. I do have my left hand, and so I can't do the normal exercises. — Shelley

ticity—especially that involving the quadriceps or adductor muscles of the inner thigh. The injections need to be repeated every 3–4 months and are expensive. In rare instances, spasticity that does not respond to standard pharmacologic management strategies requires a surgical procedure that involves cutting nerves to specific muscles.

It is important to realize that a small amount of spasticity can be helpful, especially if you experience significant weakness, because it can provide stability, or "stiffness," that may help you with standing, ambulation, and transfers.

Weakness

Muscle weakness is a common cause of walking problems such as toe drag, foot drop, *vaulting* (raising the heel on the stronger leg to make it easier to swing the weaker leg through), hip hiking, leaning over, or swinging the leg out to the side. Weakness can often be managed with appropriate exercises and assistive devices such as braces, canes, or walkers.

Weakness generally results from poor conduction in the nerves that innervate the muscles, not a problem with the muscles themselves. For this reason, exercises that involve lifting weights or repetitive movements of muscles to the point of fatigue will not strengthen the muscles. This does *not* mean that you cannot benefit from an exercise program designed for your specific needs by a PT experienced in MS care. Weak muscles that are not exercised will become even weaker. Also, the general improvement in conditioning that comes with exercise will also help to reduce weakness.

There are no medications prescribed specifically for weakness; instead, the treatment of related symptoms such as spasticity may help to improve this symptom.

Tremor

Tremor refers to an involuntary rhythmic shaking, most commonly due to the loss of myelin in the central nervous system (CNS) pathways that coordinate movement and balance. It is relatively rare with PPMS. *Intention tremor* is the most common type in MS. This occurs only during physical movement, and becomes pronounced as a person tries to grasp or reach for something, or move a hand or foot to a precise spot.

Physical or occupational therapists may be able to reduce the effects of tremor by teaching specific positions for some activities, or by exercises that stimulate the balance centers of the brain. Assistive devices such as neck or back braces/supports and weighted wrist guards and utensils, also may be helpful. Speech therapy can be helpful if your speech has been affected by tremors of the lips, tongue, or jaw.

A number of medications have been used to help manage tremor, although they are not very effective. They include oral antihistamines, which may be useful for minor tremors that are made worse by stress; beta blockers such as Inderal® (propranolol hydrochloride); medications such as Klonopin® (clonazepam) and BuSpar® (buspirone), which were originally developed as antianxiety agents, and that may help tremor by causing sedation; and Neurontin® (gabapentin) and other medications originally developed for the treatment of epilepsy, but which also have antispasticity properties.

Balance

Balance problems are not common in PPMS, but they may occur in combination with weakness and fatigue. They can result from lesions in areas of the brain involved in the control of movement; weakness, tremor, and fatigue in the muscles involved in walking; or by symptoms such as visual problems and numbness. It is possible to improve poor balance by reducing the other symptoms that contribute to it—including spasticity, weakness, and tremor—as well as by doing specific exercises.

Because balance can worsen simply as the result of being "out of condition," a basic exercise program can help improve balance at the same time that it provides general health benefits. A physical therapist with experience in PPMS can design an exercise program and teach you techniques that can help improve your balance.

OTHER SYMPTOMS THAT RESULT FROM SPINAL CORD LESIONS

In addition to the muscles of the lower limbs, damage to nerves that originate in the spinal cord also affect the organs of the lower abdomen. These include the bladder, bowel, and reproductive organs. While it might seem odd to include sexual function in the same section as bladder and bowel, this group of organs tends to be affected together because the nerves that control them are located in the same region of the spinal cord.

Bladder Dysfunction

Bladder problems are common in MS, and result from demyelination in the nervous system pathways that control the muscles of the bladder and the *sphincters* of the urinary tract that control the release of urine. The two types of bladder problems are usually referred to as "failure to store" and "failure to empty." They can usually be managed successfully once the extent of the problem is identified.

Failure-to-store problems result from a hyperactive or spastic bladder. This is the most common type of bladder dysfunction in MS. Symptoms include increased urgency and frequency of urination, incontinence, and the need to urinate during the night (*nocturia*). Changes in your diet, combined with timing urination—rather than waiting to feel the urge—may be effective. *Don't* restrict your water intake—dehydration and constipation will only add to the problem! A number of medications may be helpful, including Ditropan® and Ditropan XL® (oxybutynin), Detrol® and Detrol LA® (tolterodine tartrate), and Enablex® (darifenacin).

The failure-to-empty condition results from *flaccid* (relaxed) muscles of the bladder, such that the bladder cannot adequately contract. Symptoms include urgency followed by difficulty in starting the stream of urine, incomplete emptying, and increased frequency of urination—often the result of incomplete emptying. Urine may back up into the kidneys, which can create an even more serious problem.

The most common strategy for managing this condition is *intermittent catheterization*, usually done every few hours. In some cases, an *indwelling catheter* that remains in place for a period of time is needed, especially in people with significant disability. Medications are generally not effective for this type of bladder dysfunction, although desmopressin is often helpful in reducing the frequency of nighttime urination. Acidifying the urine with medication or cranberry juice can reduce bacteria in the bladder.

Bladder management is a toughie, because I need to maintain a certain amount of hydration to prevent fatigue. But if I drink too much, the bladder kicks in. I have some management techniques that help, such as not drinking a lot after 6:00 to make sure I get a good night's sleep.
— Tom

Sometimes, failure-to-empty bladder dysfunction results from failure of the muscles of the urinary tract system to act together in a normal pattern, so that bladder contractions to push urine out and relaxation of the sphincter to cause the release of urine do not occur together. As with the failure-to-empty bladder, either intermittent catheterization or an indwelling catheter is frequently effective, often combined with the medications used to manage failure-to-store bladder issues.

Bladder infections may occur in people with MS. They are treated with antibiotics; the specific antibiotic depends on the type of bacteria that is causing the infection.

Bowel Dysfunction

A high percentage of people with MS develop either constipation or incontinence at some time during the course of the disease. These problems can be chronic or intermittent.

Constipation is the most common bowel problem in MS; it results from lesions in the nervous system that slow the rate at which stool passes through the bowel. This causes more water to be absorbed from the gut into the body than normal, resulting in hard, dry stools. Constipation can also result from limiting the intake of fluids to minimize bladder problems, as the result of a lower activity level, or by medications taken to control other MS symptoms.

The management of constipation has three main components: diet—including at least 32 ounces a day of water or other liquids and 20–30 grams of fiber; a consistent bowel program; and the use of stool softeners, bulk formers, and other substances that increase stool bulk and stimulate more rapid passage of stool through the bowels. Laxatives are not usually recommended.

Diarrhea and fecal incontinence are relatively rare, but can be debilitating. Management primarily consists of making the stool firm and bulky, yet soft and easy to move through the bowel. Over-the-counter products such as Metamucil® are usually effective.

Sexual Difficulties

Both men and women may experience sexual difficulties in PPMS as the result of demyelination in the CNS pathways that innervate the genital areas. Problems might include loss of libido, altered genital sensation, and decreased frequency and intensity of orgasms. Men may experience difficulties with erection and ejaculation, and women may have reduced vaginal lubrication and pain during intercourse.

Many other PPMS symptoms can affect sexual function and enjoyment, including fatigue, depression, spasticity, pain, and bladder or bowel issues. Identifying and treating these symptoms may be helpful. Medications can also affect sexual function. For example, drugs that help bladder function (anticholinergic medications) can reduce vaginal secretions.

Depending upon the cause of sexual dysfunction, a variety of pharmacologic and psychosocial approaches may be helpful.

Because open communication between partners is essential to managing sexual dysfunction, counseling can be helpful. Both partners need to understand the medical and psychological issues that can affect sexuality, and be willing to work toward better communication and the possible use of alternative approaches to sexual satisfaction.

Erectile dysfunction in men might be helped by medications such as Viagra® (sildenafil), Levitra® (vardenafil), and Cialis® (tadalafil).

Medications that are directly injected into the penis, including vasodilators and papaverine, are less frequently used. Penile vacuum pumps might be an alternative if medications are not feasible.

Vaginal dryness in women can usually be managed with lubricating agents, estrogen-containing vaginal preparations, or topical creams. Spasticity and pain during intercourse may be helped by muscle relaxants.

SYMPTOMS THAT RESULT PRIMARILY FROM LESIONS IN THE BRAIN AND BRAINSTEM

Although PPMS is primarily a spinal cord disease, it is not *just* a spinal cord disease. Lesions of the brain and brainstem (an area between the brain proper and the spinal cord) do occur. These lesions result in symptoms that are similar to those experienced by many people with RRMS, including visual difficulties, speech and swallowing problems, dizziness and vertigo, cognitive difficulties, and emotional symptoms such as depression and anxiety. These issues are considered next, except for depression and anxiety, which are discussed in Chapter 8.

Cognitive Changes

Cognitive dysfunction probably affects about 25 percent of people with PPMS, in contrast to well over 50 percent in people with RRMS and SPMS. Depression, anxiety, stress, and fatigue all can affect cognitive functioning. Fatigue can particularly challenge your ability to sustain challenging mental tasks.

Symptomatic treatments and rehabilitation can help improve PPMS-related cognitive changes. To date, the most promising medications are antifatigue agents and medications used to treat Alzheimer's disease, but additional studies are needed to determine their true usefulness.

Cognitive problems in PPMS can be described as a reduction in "mental sharpness." The major areas of cognition that can be impaired include what are termed *complex attention* and *executive functions.* Complex attention involves such functions as multitasking, the speed with which information can be processed, learning and memory, and perceptual skills. Executive functions include problem solving, organizational skills, the ability to plan, and word finding.

A neuropsychological evaluation can pinpoint exactly what cognitive functions are affected and to what degree. This involves a series of tests designed to assess one or more specific cognitive changes, and to identify strengths as well as weaknesses. A neuropsychologist who has specialized training in the diagnosis and assessment of cognitive problems most often performs these evaluations.

Cognitive rehabilitation includes therapies that attempt to improve impaired abilities, such as memory or attention, by using various types of exercises or practice drills, and those designed to improve everyday functions by using strategies that "work around" impaired abilities. The frequency with which mood is improved by comprehensive cognitive rehabilitation suggests that mood—especially depression—may benefit most from this treatment approach. Improved mood can have positive effects on cognitive functioning. Also, remember that cognitive changes do not happen in a vacuum and cannot be addressed without considering your emotions and home and work environments.

Speech and Swallowing

A wide variety of speech and swallowing difficulties may occur with PPMS, depending on the areas in the brain where demyelination occurs. These problems are usually considered together, because they both tend to result from damage in the nerves that control the muscles of the torso, neck, jaw, tongue, cheeks and lips. They include spasticity, tremor, or weakness in the muscles involved in producing speech or controlling swallowing and respiration, or from a lack of muscle coordination. Speech and language pathologists manage both types of problem.

Speech

Speech difficulties result from damage to the areas of the brain that control language, speech production, swallowing, breathing, and cognition. This can range from mild difficulties to severe problems that make it difficult to speak and be understood.

The most common speech problems seen in MS are *dysarthria* and *dysphonia*. Dysarthria can involve a loss of volume (loudness) control, an unnatural emphasis on words or sentences, and a slowed rate of speaking. Dysphonia changes the *quality* of speech, such as giving a breathless quality to the voice or producing speech that sounds harsh.

A speech and language pathologist can assess the difficulties involved and possibly help improve speech patterns, pronunciation, and oral communication with exercises to strengthen and improve the muscles involved in the production of speech, and help improve breathing through relaxation of the affected muscles. If these strategies are not sufficient, many assistive devices are available to improve communication, ranging from alphabet cards to computers that speak to the user.

No medications are available specifically for improving speech. However, medications that relieve other symptoms, such as spasticity, may provide some improvement.

Swallowing

Swallowing is a complex process that involves chewing, then moving food to the back of the mouth and down through the esophagus (throat) into the stomach. Depending on lesion pattern, one or more of these processes might be affected. A speech/swallowing evaluation will determine the source of the problem and how to manage it to ensure that swallowing is safe, so that food does not enter the airway and lungs, where it can cause aspiration pneumonia. It will also focus on ensuring that food and fluid intake is sufficient for optimal health.

If safe swallowing techniques are not sufficient, in rare instances a feeding tube might need to be inserted directly into the stomach. This is a quick, safe procedure. People can still eat and drink as much they are able, using the tube as a backup to ensure adequate nutritional intake.

Visual Problems

The visual problems that are often among the first symptoms of relapsing remitting MS (RRMS) are relatively rare in PPMS. When they do occur, they can include *optic neuritis*, an inflammation of the optic nerve located behind the eye; *nystagmus*, or uncontrolled eye movements; or *diplopia* or double vision.

If visual problems persist, an ophthalmologist who specializes in low vision can provide assistive vision devices that include magnification and computer modifications, and also help design a variety of helpful strategies for managing your daily activities.

Dizziness and Vertigo

Vertigo, or the sensation of spinning, might result from lesions in those brain areas that coordinate balance. If changes in head position are a component of vertigo, a PT can develop an exercise program to help reduce the effects of positional changes.

Mild vertigo may be controlled with antihistamine such as Benadryl® (diphenhydramine) Antivert® (meclizine), or Dramamine® (dimenhydrinate), which was originally used to treat the vertigo associated with motion sickness. Scopolamine was developed to treat motion sickness and its associated vertigo, and it also might be effective; scopolamine is applied as a transdermal patch. Benzodiazepines such as Valium® (diazepam), Klonopin® (clonazepam), and Serax® (oxazepam) decrease activity in those areas of the nervous system that control the inner ear, and they may be useful in controlling vertigo.

GENERAL ISSUES

Sleep Disturbances

Sleep problems are common in PPMS, and may result from a variety of symptoms such as spasticity, urinary frequency, pain, depression, or anxiety, as well as from medications used to manage symptoms of the disease. Sleep apnea also can occur in MS. This can lead to a vicious cycle in which symptoms disturb sleep, and the lack of needed sleep worsens a variety of symptoms, such as fatigue. Addressing these problems can go a long way toward improving your sleep. Some sleep disorders are thought to be directly related to MS, so be sure to discuss this with your MS neurologist.

One of the most effective strategies to improve sleep is to develop good sleep habits. Some fairly simple changes can help enormously to ensure a good night's sleep. They include:

- ▶ **Keep a regular schedule:** Go to bed and get up at the same time every day, including weekends. This will help your body adjust to a normal sleep pattern.
- ▶ **Don't drink a lot of fluids in the evening:** To minimize nighttime trips to the bathroom, reduce fluid intake after 6 p.m.
- ▶ **Don't use the bedroom to watch TV or read:** Use it only for sleeping and sex.

▶ **Don't exercise in the evening:** Other than slow stretching to manage spasticity, do your exercise program earlier in the day.

▶ **Experiment with meditation tapes:** These and other relaxation-oriented approaches can improve the amount and quality of sleep.

Although the occasional use of sleep medications might be helpful, avoid the long-term use of sleeping pills. They lose their effectiveness quickly, are potentially addictive, and do not provide a normal night's sleep. Over-the-counter Benadryl and Benadryl-containing products may be helpful, but they should not be used on a regular basis.

Pain

PPMS can be associated with a variety of symptoms characterized as painful. In addition to the types of pain experienced by everyone—with or without MS—some types of pain are directly related to the MS process itself, while others result from physical effects of MS, such as stress on joints.

When pain is the result of demyelination of pain pathways in the brain and spinal cord, it is often described as a grinding, gnawing, or burning sensation, mostly in the legs and feet, and sometimes the trunk. This type of pain, called a *dysesthesia*, is most often treated with drugs originally developed as antiseizure medications, including Neurontin® (gabapentin), Tegretol® (carbamazepam), Lyrica® (pregabalin), or Keppra® (levetiracetam); antianxiety agents such as Valium® (diazepam) and Klonopin® (clonazepam); or antidepressants such as Elavil® (amitriptyline), Cymbalta® (duloxetine hydrochloride), or Pamelor® (nortriptyline).

Secondary pain results from MS-related problems such as urinary tract infection, pressure sores, poorly managed spasticity, poor sitting posture, problems with balance, or ill-fitting assistive devices, such as braces on the lower extremities.

Trigeminal neuralgia is a lightning-like stabbing pain in the face caused by damage to the trigeminal nerve that innervates the face. It is treated with anticonvulsant agents such as Neurontin® (gabapentin), Tegretol® (carbamazepine), or Dilantin® (phenytoin).

Lhermitte's sign is caused by damage to the cervical spinal cord. It is a brief, tingling or electric-type pain that occurs when the neck is bent forward. It moves from the head down the spine, and usually lasts for less than a second. It might go away without treatment as inflammation decreases with treatment or time. A soft neck collar can prevent the forward movement that triggers the pain, and medications such as anticonvulsants may help prevent the pain itself.

A variety of types of pain are responsive to *complementary* and *alternative medicine* strategies, including acupuncture, acupressure, guided imagery, biofeedback, yoga, and tai chi. Medicinal cannabis may be helpful, but potential cognitive problems must be considered. Low-dose naltrexone (LDN) has received a lot of attention, but has not been adequately studied.

SYMPTOMS ASSOCIATED WITH ADVANCED PPMS

The term *advanced MS* refers to people who may have significantly impaired mobility, spend extended periods of time in bed or a wheelchair, and experience more intense problems associated with some of the symptoms already discussed, such as bladder issues.

Skin Care

Most people take their skin for granted. However, skin is an organ that performs essential services for our bodies, just as much as the liver or kidneys. It has four major functions: protection from trauma and infection, sensory communication with the CNS, temperature and fluid regulation, and fat and water storage.

Lack of proper skin care can lead to serious problems in people with PPMS, because skin breakdown can result from the continual pressure caused by sitting or lying for extended periods, diminished strength, altered

Luckily, I haven't had a pressure sore because I can feel, but there have been times when I haven't paid attention and then I have to spend two weeks, three weeks in bed to clear up what might be starting as a pressure sore. — Shelley

sensation, muscle spasms, or a loss of bowel and bladder control that results in skin irritation.

Skin breakdown occurs when unrelieved pressure squeezes the tiny blood vessels that supply the skin with nutrients and oxygen. With time, the tissue dies, resulting in the formation of a *pressure sore*, also referred to as a *pressure ulcer* or a *bedsore*. These sores may be mild and involve only minor skin reddening, or they may be severe, with deep craters down to muscle and bone. *Skin reddening that disappears after pressure is applied and then removed is normal and not a pressure sore.* Infection in the skin or underlying bone is a serious problem.

Some basic guidelines for skin care, especially if you use a wheelchair or spend significant time in bed, are:

▶ Inspect the skin at least once a day, paying particular attention to areas such as the base of the spine, hips, and heels, where the underlying bone is close to the skin.

▶ Keep skin clean by regular bathing.

▶ Prevent dry skin with a good moisturizer to prevent cracking.

▶ Do not remain in the same position for more than an hour; optimally, you should reposition every 15 minutes.

▶ Report any persistent irritation promptly to your doctor or nurse.

▶ Clean the skin if it is soiled or wet from urine and pat dry. As soon as possible, cleanse the skin with a no-rinse cleanser and apply a durable barrier product.

▶ People who use a wheelchair need an air cushion or other type of cushion designed to relieve pressure. When in bed, use pillows or wedges to keep your knees or ankles from touching each other.

▶ Be sure your bed provides optimal positioning and support. To be effective, support surfaces must distribute body weight evenly over the entire body.

Respiratory Care

Areas in the brainstem control breathing. Lesions in these areas can lead to weakness in the muscles used for breathing. This in turn causes respiration to become labored. Pneumonia can occur when this is combined with decreased mobility, and swallowing difficulties can cause food particles to enter the lung.

Problems might begin slowly, possibly as a gradual increase in coughing when eating or drinking, or suddenly, as a total obstruction of the airway while eating solid food. Some medications that cause drowsiness can affect the ability to swallow, and aspiration pneumonia can result. Needless to say, if you smoke, STOP NOW!

Knowing the signs and symptoms of respiratory involvement is important to avoid a crisis. A carepartner or caregiver should pay careful attention to the following signs that a respiratory problem might be developing:

- ▶ Is breathing quiet, clear, and unlabored? Is the number of respirations in the normal range of 16 to 20 per minute?
- ▶ If any medication makes the person sleepy or lessens the number or depth of respirations, do not give him anything to eat or drink until he is more alert.
- ▶ Encourage the person to take 10 deep breaths every hour to keep the lungs clear.
- ▶ Eliminate any foods that appear to cause chewing, swallowing, or choking problems; change the diet to include either soft or blended foods; and do not include anything that requires much chewing. Have the person sit as much as possible, so that he or she can swallow with less difficulty. All family members who provide hands-on care should take a course in CPR and learn the Heimlich maneuver.
- ▶ Keep anyone who is sick away—especially those with respiratory infections. If a caregiver or family member has a cold and must be in the same room, he should wear a mask. Everyone in the house-

hold should receive an annual flu shot, and the pneumonia vaccine, as recommended—usually once every 10 years or so.

▶ Contact your physician or nurse if mucous from the mouth or nose is not clear, fever develops, or coughing becoming more frequent, because these can be signs of infection.

Urinary Tract and Bladder Issues

People with PPMS commonly require *intermittent catheterization*. This can be done by the person with the disease or by a carepartner.

If this is not sufficient, an *indwelling catheter* might be needed, either on a short- or long-term basis. Because urinary tract infections (UTIs) are fairly common with an indwelling catheter, these catheters should only be used after a combination of medications and intermittent catheterization has been tried. An indwelling catheter might also be the right solution if incontinence is contributing to the development of a pressure sore. Whatever the reason for using an indwelling catheter, it should be changed regularly, most commonly every 30 days, and more often if infection remains a problem.

Osteoporosis

We usually associate osteoporosis with middle-aged or older women. However, it is a serious problem for anyone with limited mobility who cannot do sufficient weight-bearing exercise to maintain optimal bone structure. Many people with PPMS have taken steroids, which is also a serious risk factor for developing osteoporosis.

If you have not yet had a bone-density test, you should have one now. Be sure to take a reasonable amount of calcium and vitamin D—ask your physician for the recommended dose. If early-stage bone loss is present—called *osteopenia*—or you have any level of osteoporosis, your physician will probably order one of the several medications now available to slow bone loss.

6

Technology and Adaptations That Can Make Life with Primary Progressive Multiple Sclerosis Easier to Manage

The term *assistive technology* refers to a wide variety of tools and technology that can help you modify your environment to maximize your mobility, safety, and independence. Many useful devices are available. They can be acquired as originally manufactured, or modified or customized. A physical or occupational therapist (PT or OT) can familiarize you with what is available and help you to select the right items.

Many inexpensive, low-tech items can be extremely useful and help support independence. These include reachers, Velcro® closures on clothing, nonskid bowls, and built-up handles. Other issues are more complex, such as selecting the correct mobility aid.

MOBILITY AIDS
Aids to Assist Your Ability to Walk
Ankle-Foot Orthoses

An ankle-foot orthosis (AFO) is a brace worn around the lower leg and foot that supports the ankle and holds the foot and ankle in a flexed position. Many people find this simple device very helpful to counter *foot drop*, in which lifting the foot is difficult or the ankle and toes are unable to lift upward.

Functional electrical stimulation (FES) may be an alternative to an AFO. It involves a device that sends low-level electrical impulses to the peroneal nerve, which signals the leg muscles to lift the foot. This might not be effective for everyone with PPMS, depending on how other muscles and nerves in the hip and leg are affected.

Canes

Even if an AFO is helpful, a cane might be needed to provide extra stability, especially if balance is a problem. Many types of canes and walking sticks are available, but the most popular for comfort and stability are those with palm-grip or cushioned handles.

Forearm Crutches

Lightweight forearm (Lofstrand or Canadian) crutches might be needed if balance and weakness are more advanced than can be adequately compensated for by a cane. They provide greater stability and require less strength, and either one or two might be used.

Walkers

A walker is a good choice for people with more advanced balance and endurance issues, but who are able to walk because they provide free-standing stability. Depending on your specific needs, walkers are available with and without wheels, and can include hand brakes, seats, baskets, trays, and other useful add-ons.

Wheelchairs: Finding the Right One for Your Needs

If canes, crutches, and walkers are not adequate, you may need a wheelchair, either manually propelled or motorized. A wide variety is available. Choosing the correct wheelchair is an important decision, as it will become your "legs," and your overall comfort and function depends on making the right decision. Ask the therapist lots of questions and discuss your personal lifestyle and how you will use the chair. Hospital groups and outpatient therapy services sometimes host wheelchair clinics where, with a doctor's referral, a person needing a wheelchair can be seen by the therapist and rehab supplier in the same location. This provides an opportunity to discuss the best possible options with experts. As with any major purchase, you should identify the most reputable suppliers in your area.

Wheelchair specialists, usually either OTs or PTs, will consider a number of issues when selecting and customizing your chair, and might suggest visiting a wheelchair clinic to consult with an assistive technology professional or durable medical equipment (DME) provider and try out a variety of options. At this time:

▶ The chair will be individually customized to fit, taking into account leg length, the angle of knee bending that is appropriate, the correct depth and width of the seat, the kind of back that will provide optimal support, and whether features such as the ability to tilt and recline are needed.

▶ The right cushion will be selected to provide comfortable support and prevent areas of pressure. Seating experts might use pressure-mapping equipment to document the kind of cushion needed.

▶ The layout and design of your home will be analyzed to be sure the wheelchair can be used appropriately, and transportability will be discussed (car, van, and public transportation).

▶ A variety of possible chairs will be considered, focusing on how they might meet your needs over time.

MANUAL AND POWER WHEELCHAIRS. One basic decision will be whether a manual or power wheelchair is most appropriate. Many factors need to be considered, including your strength and physical condition, how much fatigue you experience, transportation options, and how you will use the chair at home and in the community. Insurance issues will also be involved, especially if it is necessary to choose a single chair to meet most of your needs. Many insurers will expect you to use the chair for a minimum of 5–7 years.

Adequate upper body strength is needed to use a manual wheelchair, and there should be only a minimal amount of fatigue when using it. A wide variety is available, most of them quite lightweight and portable. The major advantage of a manual chair is that it can fold up and fit into the trunk of a car; some have removable tires, armrests, and footrests, and can be very easily transported.

A power wheelchair might be the best option if you have more advanced mobility issues or significant fatigue. They come in many varieties and configurations, including ones that tilt or recline to relieve pressure and prevent pressure ulcers.

Now I get around with Access-A-Ride. It's a really good service. They pick you up from your starting point and take you to your destination. I go to all my appointments that way.

— Jason

SCOOTERS. Scooters are widely used by people with a range of mobility issues. They can be either three- or four-wheeled, and are most appropriate for people who can walk and don't require them full time. A scooter can greatly increase your ability to move about the home or in the community. A seating clinic with a PT or OT is advisable to help you consider all of the issues (leg room, turning radius, etc.) and options (swing-away armrests, portability, etc.) so that you get what you pay for. (Insurance companies often deny payment for a scooter if it is not needed in the home.)

DRIVING

Except for people living in cities with good, accessible public transportation and/or paratransit systems, most North Americans use their cars daily. They are an essential part of our working and social lives. If PPMS makes it difficult to drive, a variety of options can help you maintain mobility.

Adapted driving is not for everyone. For example, symptoms such as poor vision, severe hand tremors, and cognitive difficulties make driving an unworkable option.

An adapted van is the most common vehicle used by people with PPMS. A variety of situations must be considered, depending on your ability and inclination: Will you be driving while in a wheelchair? Entering as a passenger? Or, transferring from your wheelchair to a regular seat? Options include lowered-floor minivans, wheelchair lifts, and rear-entry kneeling vans. The van's controls can be adapted with a joystick or—for people with more advanced levels of disability—with other options. These modifications do not prevent other drivers from using the van.

Mechanisms for driving while using a power wheelchair include headrests with driving controls, tongue and cheek switches, a specialized touch pad, and more. A creative and experienced vendor and an OT who is a driving specialist can help you make the best decision. For more information about local vendors, contact the National MS Society or the MS Association of America. The National Mobility Equipment Dealers Association (NMEDA, www.nmeda.org; 800-833-0427) can help connect you with companies in your area that work with people with disabilities to meet their transportation needs.

Most auto-makers offer rebates if you are buying a new vehicle that needs adaptation. Talk with your dealership or the National MS Society about rebate programs. Another option is to purchase a used vehicle. The cost is significantly less, and they often come with substantial warranties. Search the Internet for companies that rent wheelchair-accessible vans and sell them at a reduced price.

Funding for wheelchair-adapted vehicles can be hard to obtain, but groups such as the National MS Society, Centers for Independent Living, veterans organizations, faith-based organizations, and fraternal groups might be able to help you get the funds you need. In some states, Medicaid covers lift systems. Every state has an assistive technology financial loan program. You can find this information at: www.resna.org/AFTAP/index.html or by calling 703-524-6686. These programs provide low-cost loans to enable people with disabilities to obtain equipment and make home modifications.

AUGMENTATIVE COMMUNICATION DEVICES

PPMS does not usually take away the ability to communicate. If it does, *augmentative communication devices* can help you communicate more easily and effectively.

Manual communication boards, which have no moving parts, are an inexpensive and practical way to communicate. A toothbrush, portrayed as a photograph, symbol, and/or printed words represents the idea that the user wants to brush her teeth; she simply points or gestures to the symbol. Word or letter boards also can be created to allow the user to point to and spell out words or everyday phrases.

A higher-technology approach includes augmentative speech and amplification devices. Computer software can convert text to speech and recognize speech (even slurred speech). Modifications can be made to the keyboard and mouse, and head and eye control systems are available.

HOME MODIFICATIONS

If you or a loved one has difficulty navigating in the home, you will need to consider modifications. Depending on your home's structure and layout and the level of disability, only minor physical changes may be necessary. In other cases, major changes will be needed. We refer you to the booklet *Accessible Home Design* for suggestions.

One very helpful option to increasing your accessibility to all areas of your home is an *electronic aid for daily living unit* (EADL), formerly called an *environmental control unit* (ECU). This unit can be located by the bedside to operate the TV, telephone, lights, call system, and other devices. Voice-activated models are also available. This type of device promotes independence and means that family carepartners may need to be called upon for help less often.

Adaptations for Multi-Story Homes

If you live in a multi-story home, moving your bedroom to the main floor might be a simple, reasonable solution. To provide full access to your home, stairlifts and residential elevators are very helpful. The ability to transfer and maintain good sitting balance are required to use a stairlift. Elevators specifically designed for home use include the Minivator, a small elevator for use when space is limited.

Elevators and stairlifts can be expensive. Veterans may be able to obtain at least partial funding from the Office of Veterans Affairs (VA). Some towns and states provide funding for home modifications. Contact your state department of social services, a local independent living center, the National MS Society, or the MS Association of America for funding ideas. It might also be possible to buy some equipment secondhand, but be sure you are getting it from a reliable source and that it is appropriate for your needs. Try it out before buying to make sure it works properly, and work with a professional to ensure that it addresses your specific needs and the layout of your home.

Kitchen Adaptations

A wide variety of adaptations and equipment can be helpful if fatigue or weakness affects navigating in the kitchen and preparing food. Simple items such as reachers can help you get things off high shelves, but a simple rearrangement of where things are stored might be all that's needed. An OT can help you choose the right equipment and suggest changes that will make your kitchen more user-friendly.

More extensive renovations might include making all kitchen equipment accessible at a lower height for a person who uses a wheelchair, but this would normally be done only as part of a major home modification or if you are building a new home.

Bathroom Adaptations

Many devices and equipment can improve bathroom comfort and safety, including bathtub seats or benches, transfer seats, handheld showers, wheel-in showers, and shower chairs. Low-tech items that can make bathing easier include soap-on-a-rope and washcloth mitts. If bathing must take place in bed, a bath-in-bed unit or a shower-any-where portable shower can be very helpful. See Appendix 2 for catalogs and websites that provide this kind of equipment.

Portable toilet chair features such as adjustable height, removable arms, seat lifts, and the ability to double as a shower chair are good options to look for. A variety of bedpans and urinals can be used for toileting in bed.

Home Automation

Major advances have occurred in the area of wireless environmental control systems, by which major components of your home's environment—lighting, climate control, doors, phone, etc.—can be controlled by voice activation or with a small remote from a single location. Many user-friendly products do not require a specialist to install. An OT might be a good resource when beginning to explore these options; www.homecontrols.com is a catalog supplier of this type of device.

OTHER ASSISTIVE DEVICES

Many products are available for just having fun! Large screen TVs can help people with poor vision enjoy TV and movies. Low-tech items such as playing card holders or books on tape can make card playing and reading relaxing and fun again. A wheelchair camera mount can allow a person who cannot hold a camera to enjoy photography as a hobby. Wheelchairs with special tires can be used on sand or rough terrain, opening up possibilities for outings to the beach or woods, and several gardening adaptations are also available.

Many travel agencies, travel guides, and other resources are available for people with disabilities. Many cruise lines and hotels provide wheelchair-accessible rooms. An OT or PT can help you brainstorm ideas to make your trip more enjoyable, such as traveling with a portable bed rail to make bed mobility and transfers easier.

Wellness and Primary Progressive Multiple Sclerosis: An Attainable Goal

Some of the material in this chapter is based on a National MS Society publication on wellness, available at www.nationalmssociety.org/living-with-multiple-sclerosis/getting-the-care-you-need/my-life-my-ms-my-decisions/index.aspx.

WHAT IS WELLNESS WHEN YOU HAVE PPMS?

Can you really achieve "wellness" while living with primary progressive multiple sclerosis (PPMS)? Absolutely—it is not only possible; it is a *necessary* part of having good overall quality of life! Wellness means achieving a healthy balance between mind, body, and spirit that produces an overall feeling of well-being. Making the most of your physical and emotional health will enhance your quality of life by allowing you to do those things that you really want to do and achieve a satisfying balance of self-care, play, and work, or other productive activities.

MS isn't the only thing in my life. I want to take care of myself to the best of my ability from an MS standpoint, but I also want to prevent other diseases. What a shame it would be to develop a disease that I could have prevented. — Tom

Even though you have PPMS, you are as susceptible to the same wide variety of medical conditions as anyone else. It is important to take charge of your overall health—all those guidelines about healthy eating, getting exercise, not smoking, and getting regular checkups apply to *YOU*! In addition to the specialists who manage your MS, you should see your primary care physician regularly to receive the preventive care you need. This is especially important because other medical conditions can alter the symptoms of PPMS and your ability to function optimally. If you smoke—stop NOW. Millions of people have, and you can, too. Smoking worsens some MS symptoms and increases the risks of complications from MS.

When I decided not to return to work, I felt like I needed to step back and emotionally disconnect from years of a career and begin to focus on myself and my health issues and how I was going to make my life with my family more rich and fulfilling.
— Kathy

Screening tests, such as a periodic colonoscopy or mammogram, can find diseases early when they are easier to treat. We strongly suggest that you review the document "Preventive Care Recommendations for Adults with MS," which can be accessed on the National MS Society website at: www.nationalmssociety.org/brochures. It provides guidelines for regular health checkups as well as general health and safety recommendations.

The road to wellness should be viewed as an ongoing *process*—a journey that you will continue to follow as you integrate new behaviors into your life. It is equally important to address health promotion and disease prevention strategies; develop a strong support network of family and friends; have satisfying work and leisure activities, and a meaningful place in the community; and pay adequate attention to your inner self.

I want to enjoy what I can and not dwell on what I can't do. Otherwise, I've given away more of my life to MS than it deserves. — Shelley

Wellness is much more than physical fitness, but being as fit as possible in the presence of PPMS is essential to making all the other components of wellness possible—emotional, spiritual, and social. Achieving physical fitness does not need to involve aggressive strength training, aerobics, or calisthenics. A sensible, gentle program based on *your* specific needs and abilities will yield major benefits.

EXERCISE AS A COMPONENT OF PHYSICAL FITNESS

Regular exercise is important for everyone, with or without PPMS. It can give you the strength and energy to do those things that are most important to you. Although symptoms such as weakness, spasticity, or fatigue may make exercising on a routine basis more difficult, regular activity will enhance your physical and psychological well-being. Exercise has a number of beneficial effects, including:

▶ Maintaining or improving joint flexibility and muscle strength
▶ Maintaining or improving the function of the heart, blood vessels, and respiratory system
▶ Helping to prevent osteoporosis
▶ Maximizing energy levels and reducing fatigue
▶ Relaxing the body and reducing stress
▶ Reducing the incidence of falls
▶ Improving mood
▶ Reducing any tendency to constipation
▶ Assisting with weight control
▶ Promoting an inner sense of achievement and well-being

Any exercise program should be designed with the input of a physical therapist (PT) or other appropriate health care professional. Check with your local National MS Society chapter, many of which sponsor exercise programs or can refer you to local classes.

I can't strengthen the muscles that are weakened directly from the MS. But I can strengthen the ones that have been weakened because of inactivity. —Tom

Whatever physical activity program you choose, it is important to stay with it. Seek out new ways to maintain your interest, so that fitness becomes a way of life, and think about how determination, motivation, and self-discipline can help keep you on track.

A great way to stay more physically active is to make it part of your daily life. If you enjoy walking, consider incorporating more walking into everyday errands or social activities. A recumbent tricycle with a carrying basket could be a great way to shop for groceries, as long as you can ride on a safe street or bike path. By involving friends and family members in physical activity, you might even become a role model for those around you.

Stretching and Range of Motion Exercises

Begin any workout with a basic stretching routine. Stretching on its own can provide significant benefits, especially to reduce spasticity. You should not feel pain while stretching—or during any part of your exercise routine. Do not force any part of your body or push beyond your comfort limit. If you are unaware of some muscles because of numbness, tingling, or functional loss, stretch lightly. *Remember that stretching is about slow, controlled movements.* Moving too quickly or forcefully can result in injury. If you experience any pain or discomfort during exercise, stop immediately and check with your PT or other health care professional before doing that exercise again.

Stretching will help maintain range of motion in your joints, which is important in maintaining overall joint health, as well as preventing *contractures*, a situation such as "frozen shoulder" or a knee that won't straighten. We recommend the stretching section in *Multiple Sclerosis: A Self-Care Guide to Wellness.*

Aquatics

Aquatics—exercise done in water—is often recommended for people with MS. Aquatics can help improve strength and flexibility, while avoiding overheating. The recommended pool temperature is 85 degrees or less—especially if the surrounding area is hot and humid. Because water reduces the effects of gravity, the resulting buoyancy will help you achieve a greater range of motion. Chest-high water also provides support, enabling many people to stand and maintain their balance while exercising with much less effort than on land. The resistance that water provides can also help strengthen muscles.

Yoga

Yoga involves breathing exercises and a range of stretches that increase flexibility and release tension. Many National MS Society chapters, community centers, and health clubs have yoga classes. Some of the movements may be easy, while others may be inappropriate or need practice or modification. Alert your yoga instructor to the potential need for an individual evaluation. Books and videos for "gentle yoga" routines are available.

Tai Chi

Tai chi involves deep breathing, slow gentle movements, and relaxation. As a conditioning regimen, it is considered a gentler form of exercise than yoga. Many of the positions can be done while sitting.

Pilates

Pilates exercise teaches awareness of breathing and alignment of the spine, and aims to strengthen muscles in the body's core—the deep torso muscles. Students are instructed to perform every exercise with the utmost control of all body parts, to avoid injury and produce positive results. The number or intensity of repetitions is less important than proper form to ensure safe and effective results.

Although it is safe to exercise when you have PPMS, it is also important to listen to your body! Try to be realistic. Know your limits, and remember that it's okay to rest, to take a day off, or to do only 15 minutes instead of your regular 30. Overexertion and heat during exercise can *temporarily* aggravate MS symptoms. Despite this, a well-designed exercise regimen has many benefits, while a continued lack of physical activity will lead to further deconditioning or general sense of weakness.

My philosophy is, if I can move it, I move it. And if I can't move it, I'll have somebody else move it for me. Range of motion is very, very important for people who cannot move their own joints and muscles, just to maintain mobility and flexibility.
— Tom

Any activity that gets your body moving is beneficial. It might involve a formal exercise program—but it doesn't have to. Reluctant exercisers will get a psychological lift just from taking control of this important component of good health. Physical activity releases the "fight-or-flight" *adrenaline* hormone, which revs up the body and mind for action, as well as *endorphins*, known for their mood-elevating and painkilling power. Thus, exercise leads to the sense of well-being that is so important in our lives.

NUTRITION

A sensible diet is a critical part of living with PPMS. While no magic foods or combination of foods and supplements has proven to affect MS or its symptoms over the long term, a poor diet will do nothing to make you feel better while dealing with the symptoms of PPMS.

Good health has a lot to do with what you put on your plate at every meal, so diet is an area where you can be in control of your health. Eating for good health is as simple as A-B-C: **A**im for fitness, **B**uild a healthy base, and **C**hoose sensibly.

▶ **Aim for fitness:** Make achieving a healthy weight your target. There are many reasons why you might gain or lose weight, but the things you need to do to control your weight are the same as for everyone else. Physical activity and good nutrition are perfect partners in managing your weight.

▶ **Build a healthy base:** Translating good nutrition to your dinner table takes planning, attention, and some innovation. Let the U.S. Department of Agriculture's Food Guide Pyramid provide a starting point. The Pyramid will help you choose a balanced plan that is right for you. The *MyPyramid* plan can be accessed at www.mypyramid.gov.

Grains, fruits, and vegetables should be the foundation of your diet. Choices from these groups are rich in vitamins, minerals, carbohydrates, and other nutrients. Most of the foods in this group help create a feeling of fullness and satisfaction that will quiet the urge for unhealthy snacks. Many people find that eating smaller meals more often is a good way to manage their weight by controlling the total number of calories they consume.

If I want to get out and spread mulch around, I just do it differently. I make sure I'm close to things I can hold onto, and use a rake or a shovel or something to help me walk. But I pretty much do everything I've always done.
— Kathy

▶ **Choose sensibly:** There are many ways to build a personal pyramid, and lots of room for choice. When in doubt, go easy on fat, sugar, and sodium. The Nutrition Fact Label on food products can be a useful tool to do this.

Trim the fat from your diet—especially saturated fat and trans fats. This not only cuts calories, but it might decrease your risk of developing disorders such as heart disease and stroke. Use vegetable oils instead of solid fats such as butter and hard margarine. Choose fat-free or low-fat dairy products and lean meats. Trim the skin from poultry.

Nutritional strategies can be extremely helpful in managing some of the symptoms of PPMS, fatigue being perhaps the best example. When combined with a good exercise strategy, you should see a significant improvement in managing this difficult symptom.

Nutrition and Fatigue

People with MS can develop fatigue for many reasons, as discussed in Chapter 5. Whatever its cause, fatigue can result in a decrease in appetite and general activity, as well as less interest in food preparation.

Shopping for groceries can be real a challenge. Not many of us get excited about going to the supermarket. It can be even more difficult when you are feeling fatigued. Here are some tips that can make the experience a little easier:

- ▶ Make a shopping list before you go to the store.
- ▶ Plan the shopping trip for your best time of day, and make it part of the day's physical activity plan.
- ▶ Plan your list according to the layout of the store, so that you can maximize your energy and not have to retrace your steps.
- ▶ Try to spend the major part of your time on the outside perimeter of the store. That's typically where you will find fruits, vegetables, and protein-rich foods.
- ▶ If you have difficulty carrying bags of groceries, find delivery services, shopping services, or friends and relatives who will shop from your list. A fold-up shopping cart might also be helpful.

When you cook, here are some tips to make sure your nutritional needs are met if fatigue becomes a challenge:

- ▶ If the thought of three large meals is too much, try eating five or six smaller meals.
- ▶ Keep your refrigerator and cupboards stocked with items that you use regularly, and include healthy foods that will help you resist the urge to eat low-nutrient, convenience foods.

▶ Packaged prechopped vegetables can cut down your preparation time, or once a week you can prepare veggies to refrigerate and cook later. Shredded cheese, jars of minced garlic or ginger root, sliced olives, and diced peppers save energy.

▶ Stock up on flavorful, low-fat dinners that can be quickly microwaved or heated. When you cook, try to make more than you will eat in one meal and store or freeze the rest.

▶ The process of preparing a meal and cleaning up afterward can be time-consuming and not exactly fun, so consider the following tips:

- Ask your doctor for a referral to an occupational therapist (OT) to help with kitchen adaptations that will best meet your needs. Among the items that can increase efficiency are utensils, storage systems, reaching aids, and adapted stovetops.

- Removing doors underneath cabinet countertops allows you to sit while preparing food. Just make sure any hot pipes are wrapped with insulation.

- Streamline cleanup! Paper plates can be a lifesaver when energy is low. Enlist family and friends as extra hands, and save your energy for socializing after the meal.

Eating out or ordering in are always good options if you just haven't had time to get to the store or don't want to deal with fixing a meal. But it can be easy to make poor choices. Consider these ideas:

▶ Keep a stack of menus from places that deliver healthy meals.

▶ When eating out, think ahead about what you will order and avoid high-calorie items.

▶ When portion sizes are large, "box-up" half the meal before beginning to eat.

ENERGY CONSERVATION

Fatigue can affect the quality of your daily life, making it essential to adopt energy-saving, effective strategies such as:

▶ **Set priorities:** List your activities, rank them in order of importance, then choose those that are most appealing.

▶ **Delegate tasks:** Identify tasks that other people can do for you. Remember that being independent does not mean doing everything independently; it also means knowing how to get help when you need it.

▶ **Simplify and eliminate tasks:** Consider which tasks can be eliminated and which could be simplified or done differently.

▶ **Plan ahead:** Improve how you organize the day's activities. Plan your movements around the house. Put everything you need for a particular activity in one place, and plan what will be needed during the week. Place a bulletin board or dry-erase board in a central location, so that family members can add to the shopping list. Plan your travel outside your home, bring a list for easier shopping, write down errands in a date book, and see whether errands can be combined.

▶ **Balance your schedule:** The key is to prevent exhaustion by knowing your limits and abilities. Develop a realistic schedule for your activities for the week, and then plan your days. Alternate periods of work and rest. Pace activities and avoid doing several things at once.

▶ **Work effectively:** Maintain good posture by sitting in a straight firm chair, making sure your lower back is well supported. At a table, make sure the height is appropriate, and face your work head-on. Don't lock your knees when standing. Lift objects by keeping them as close to the body as possible. Keep your work space well-organized. Choose practical, adapted work tools.

▶ **Analyze activities/solve problems:** First, identify a problem and determine its source. Then, brainstorm solutions and select one you think will work. Evaluate the results. If it didn't work, try one of the other solutions you brainstormed earlier. If none of your ideas are productive, consult an outside source, such as an OT.

DEALING WITH STRESS

Some people experience more symptoms during times of stress, and symptoms often seem less troubling or severe when stress is lessened. Stress is a normal part of everyday life, and it is unrealistic to think that we can eliminate it completely. However, you can learn to reduce its intensity and use it to work for, not against, you.

Stressful situations that are common with PPMS include:

▶ Uncertainty about the future
▶ Other people's reactions to your MS symptoms
▶ The need to adjust and readjust to changing abilities
▶ Financial stress and concerns about employment
▶ Loss of control due to issues such as bladder dysfunction
▶ The need to make decisions about major life changes, such as living environment, relationships, and the use of assistive devices and mobility aids

Knowing what causes or increases personal stress can be the first step in dealing with it. Make a list of the events and concerns that were the most troubling to you during the last two weeks.

Next, think how to better manage situations, so that they don't create more stress than necessary. Building a support network of people who know about your illness and the difficulties it causes can be a good first step. Talking

Some days are better than others, and every day is different. I call them hundred-dollar days, or seventy-five dollar days, or fifty-dollar days. If I'm having a hundred-dollar day, that's great. I'll do as much as I can with that hundred dollars. That's where fatigue management and energy management really comes in. It's like having a certain amount of money to spend, but if you don't spend it you can't carry it over to the next day. — Tom

My church is a great support system. People there know the situation with MS and understand it.
— *Kathy*

with others may help you see those things that cause you stress in a new light. In addition to family and friends, consider expanding your resources to include a support group—online, telephone, or face-to-face. Counseling might also be helpful.

There is no single right way to cope with stress. No one method is better or worse than any other. Strategies that might be helpful include:

- ▶ Anticipate stressful situations and how they might be handled. Are there ways to avoid the situations that cause stress, or do you need to develop ways to adjust to a stressful situation?
- ▶ Prioritize what needs to be done, and simplify your life by eliminating what's not absolutely necessary.
- ▶ Get extra sleep, especially before family gatherings or important events.
- ▶ Learn to say no. Don't do anything if you don't have the time, energy, or desire.
- ▶ Take time for the things that bring you pleasure.
- ▶ Relax a few of your standards. Ask yourself if a particular task needs to be done perfectly, or if it needs to be done at all.
- ▶ If old interests and activities become more difficult or too time-consuming, replace them with new ones that fit your current needs.

Call your local community center, the Y, the National MS Society, or the MS Association of America to find classes on stress and time management, relaxation, yoga, or tai chi. Check your local library for videos or audiotapes on stress management.

Emotional and Quality-of-Life Issues

It is easy to get caught up in the health care system and the focus on helping you manage your *physical* symptoms. Although symptom management is a crucial part of dealing with PPMS, it should never be at the expense of other areas. Many people especially neglect the emotional issues associated with PPMS, despite the fact that they are extremely common and have a huge impact on quality of life.

Common mental health issues related to PPMS include depression, anxiety, cognitive impairment, anger, and stress. Many nonmedical issues that contribute to these problems and ways of coping are discussed in detail in other chapters.

It is important to be as alert to emotional and cognitive changes as you are to physical ones. Memory problems, word-finding difficulty, slowed processing speed, mood swings, and even depression can occur in anyone. These problems require immediate attention because they can alter your ability to learn, develop strategies for dealing with problems, and manage your own self-care. Because some medications taken to manage MS symptoms or other medical problems can affect emotions and cognition, contact your physician, counselor, or nurse as soon as these side effects arise.

Some people delay seeking help for mental health concerns because they believe that needing this kind of assistance means they are "weak." However, *everyone* can benefit from help with emotional issues. Seeking assistance demonstrates purposeful action and strength.

QUALITY-OF-LIFE NEEDS

Some common symptoms experienced by people with PPMS have a tremendous effect on social patterns with friends and families. Based on feedback from people with PPMS, a "quality of life needs ladder" was identified. It includes independence and "normalcy"—things that most people take for granted, such as going places where and when they want to, dignity, and enjoying social relationships. People with PPMS tend to move down on this ladder as their disease progresses.

People with PPMS who participated in the PPMS focus groups discussed in the Introduction to this book tended to view a "good day" as one during which they were not experiencing major symptoms, felt energized, were without pain or stress, could think clearly, and were able to participate in normal activities and enjoy simply being alive and loved. On a "bad day," they focused more on symptoms—including fatigue, weakness, stress, depression, medication issues, and bowel and bladder problems. They felt a lack of human contact, and believed they had nothing to look forward to.

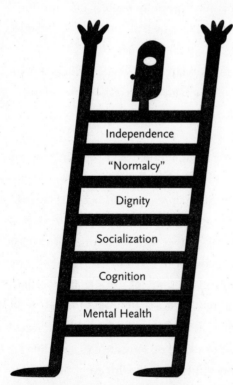

Independence

"Normalcy"

Dignity

Socialization

Cognition

Mental Health

QUALITY OF LIFE NEEDS "LADDER"

When asked what concerned them the most, people with PPMS focused on what the future would bring, how the disease would affect their relationships, worries about becoming a burden on their families, financial issues, and a general fear of the unknown.

Emotional problems are especially common at the time of diagnosis, when many people report feeling "scared and confused." Despite this, referrals to a social worker or other professional who could provide emotional support are often lacking. In addition to recommending a counselor, neurologists are encouraged to suggest that their newly diagnosed patients contact the National MS Society and the MS Association of America to learn more about PPMS and available services. Even when counseling is recommended, some people may experience difficulty accessing mental health services because of financial and insurance issues, which adds to the problems of dealing with the diagnosis.

A recurring theme among people with PPMS and their carepartners is that they need support groups specifically targeted to their needs, rather than to those of the general MS population. In response, the National MS Society is developing regional telephone support groups, pilots for which will become active in 2010.

These new programs for people with PPMS will *empower* them by providing programs, services, information, and support that focus on adapting to change and remaining functional and productive members of their families and communities.

INDEPENDENCE AND PRODUCTIVITY

One of the difficult issues that might need to be dealt with after a diagnosis of PPMS is the change from being independent to increasing dependency resulting from disabling symptoms. Assistive devices such as walkers, scooters, wheelchairs, equipment for activities of daily living, and environmental adaptations become a reality of daily life with PPMS, and it is important to remember that the appropriate use of these devices can help you continue to be independent, despite disease progression (see Chapter 6).

It is also important to remain productive and involved in daily activities. While this can be difficult, you can redefine "productivity" in relation to your own changing life. For example, you might not be able to play baseball with your children, but you can go to games to cheer them on, help with homework, and play games.

Adjusting to PPMS

The goal of emotional adjustment is to adapt to the presence of MS in your daily life. This can be a tiring process. Your emotional reactions, and those of your family members, will ebb and flow with changes in your illness. Each new symptom or change in function means that you have to readjust your plans. As discussed by Dr. Rosalind Kalb in *Multiple Sclerosis: A Guide for Families*, this requires making room for the disease without giving it any more space, time, or energy than it absolutely needs. This is easier said than done, and you might need professional help to achieve this goal.

EMOTIONAL REACTIONS TO PPMS

Each of us builds a picture of who we are over our lifetime. When this picture changes, everyone involved needs to grieve before putting the pieces together and developing a new image. Counseling can help.

As the reality of living with PPMS sinks in, typical reactions include anxiety about the future and anger that this is happening to *you*. You may experience periods of grief and loss. Every new symptom and each new medication can represent a loss of certainty and control, or the loss of a particular skill or ability.

Guilt and a feeling of loss of control are among the most common reactions to the diagnosis of PPMS. Guilt can take a variety of forms. It may be related to a real or perceived inability to fulfill your roles and responsibilities in different areas of life. You may worry that you are letting others down—especially family members—and that you are no longer contributing what you think you should be to your family. It is important that you acknowledge and deal with these emotions.

Depression

Depression affects 15–20 percent of all Americans during their lifetimes, and up to one-half of all people with MS experience episodes of depression during the course of the disease. Depression can seriously affect motivation, sleeping patterns, eating habits, and energy. Each of these can, in turn, affect your quality of life and overall well-being.

Depression can occur for a number of reasons, including:

▶ Fatigue
▶ Changes in abilities and physical status
▶ Changes in life plans
▶ Fear of rejection by family and friends
▶ Decreased self-esteem or a change in self-image
▶ MS lesions in areas of the brain that directly affect emotions
▶ Neurochemical changes in the brain that affect emotions

Although people with PPMS can become depressed at any time, certain times and experiences are associated with greater risk, including:

▶ At the time of diagnosis
▶ With increasing disability
▶ Times of transition to greater dependence, such as needing an ambulation aid or personal assistance
▶ Any major life change or loss, such as disability-related retirement

When I was diagnosed in 1980, I was relieved because I now had something that I could call my own, if you will. But that didn't last very long, because I knew that I had some kind of a disease going on in my brain and that it was going to continue to progress and make me worse. I started to grieve the loss. It wasn't that I lost anything. I mean, I wasn't able to run as well as I had previously, but I was actually projecting my loss, and I was grieving things that I hadn't even lost yet, which is kind of weird. But it was a feeling of the unknown—what's going to happen to me? — Tom

Family members are also at risk of depression during these times, especially when lifestyle changes occur and caregiving needs increase.

Depression may be relatively mild, and the support of friends and family may be all that's needed to help you get through a difficult time. For others, it is a serious problem that can last for several months or more, affecting sleep and interfering with work, family, and social relationships.

I really went through Kubler-Ross's five stages of grief— denial, anger, bargaining, and finally acceptance.
— Jason

Depression does not indicate weak character, and it is not something that needs to be hidden. It cannot be controlled or prevented by willpower or determination. In its most severe forms, it appears to be a chemical imbalance in the brain that can occur at any time, even when life is going well. It can often be alleviated by talking about the problem and by taking the appropriate medications.

How Is Clinical Depression Treated?

Supportive family, friends, and support groups might be able to help you shake off mild depression, but psychotherapy and/or antidepressant medication are usually needed to treat the condition adequately and prevent an even deeper depression from developing. Treatment should address your needs as a whole person, as well as your living situation.

Many antidepressant medications are available, but none is a "magic bullet." Some produce improvement within several days, but the full effect usually does not appear for several weeks. If no improvement occurs after 6 weeks, your doctor might increase the dose, add another medication, or prescribe a different one.

Few physicians believe that medication alone cures depression. Most recommend combining drug therapy with counseling. "Talk therapy," or *psychotherapy*, facilitates the grieving process, promotes self-esteem, and improves coping, communication, and problem-solving skills. It can be provided by psychiatrists, physicians who can prescribe

What Are the Characteristics of Clinical Depression?

The symptoms of depression are not the normal, transient "blues" that everyone experiences in response to a sad or distressing event. The hallmark of clinical depression is that the symptoms don't go away. The symptoms of a major depressive episode last at least two weeks, and they can seriously impair daily functioning. During that time, five or more of the following nine symptoms are experienced on a daily, almost round-the-clock basis. One or both of the first two is always present in a major depressive episode.

- Feeling sad or empty, or being irritable or tearful most of the day, nearly every day
- A loss of interest or pleasure in most activities
- Significant weight loss or gain, or a decrease or increase in appetite
- Sleeping too much or an inability to sleep
- Physical restlessness or slowed movement that is observed by others
- Ongoing fatigue or loss of energy
- Feeling personally worthless or guilty without appropriate cause
- A diminished ability to concentrate or make decisions
- Recurrent thoughts of death or suicide, or planning suicide

If you experience five or more of these symptoms consistently for more than two weeks, seek immediate professional intervention and treatment. Acknowledging that a problem exists and seeking aid is the most important thing you can do.

medication as well as counseling. Psychologists, psychiatric nurses, licensed professional counselors, certified social workers, and other qualified nonphysicians also provide counseling and work with physicians to select and monitor medication if needed.

Talk therapy can address a current crisis; it might be supportive and focus on finding ways to cope, or it might involve in-depth exploration with the goal of helping you develop greater self-awareness. The form depends on your specific needs, which may change over time. Family and carepartners might also be involved.

Therapy can be supplemented by participating in a self-help group. Being with others who have similar problems can be reassuring, and it can help you to realize that your reactions are reasonable and understandable. Ask the National MS Society about self-help group programs in your area.

> I get into what I call a depression/anger cycle. It might be due to the MS. I mean, that's part of MS— an organic depression as a direct result of the disease process or cognitive involvement, whatever. Some days I get frozen in depression . . . I can't make a decision, what to eat or what to do. I know how to undo it, it's just to do something and make some kind of a decision. — Tom

Antidepressant Medications

Antidepressant medications can help manage depression. They act by making natural chemicals called *neurotransmitters* more available to the brain and restoring its chemical balance. These include the classes of drugs termed *selective serotonin re-uptake inhibitors* (SSRIs), such as Prozac® (fluoxetine), Zoloft® (Sertraline), Paxil® (paroxetine), Celexa® (citalopram), and Lexapro® (escitalopram); *selective serotonin and norepinephrine reuptake inhibitors* (SNRIs) such as Cymbalta® (duloxetine hydrochloride), Serzone® (nefazodone), Wellbutrin® (bupropion), and Remeron® (mirtazapine); and *tricyclic antidepressants* such as Elavil® (amitriptyline), Tofranil® (imipramine), or Pamelor® (nortriptyline).

Wellness Strategies

A number of wellness strategies can improve the symptoms of depression, including exercise, nutrition, and good sleep habits. Any regular fitness program will improve your physical and mental health. The *endorphins* released during physical activity induce feelings of well-being and relaxation. Depression can be associated with poor food choices and overeating, or with a reduced appetite. Both are harmful to your overall wellness and health. Tune in to how mood affects your food choices. Chapter 7 discusses wellness strategies in detail.

Anxiety

Like depression, anxiety is a common response to living with PPMS. It is characterized by worry, agitation, apprehension, and other symptoms that can include impaired concentration, disrupted sleep, irritability, restlessness, muscle tension, excessive fatigability (which can easily be confused with MS fatigue), and panic attacks.

Anxiety is usually treated with a combination of medication and psychotherapy. Some forms of depression are accompanied by symptoms of anxiety.

One of the best ways to manage anxiety is with a program of gentle stretching, breathing, and movement, combined with medication as needed. *Yoga* can be adapted for people with PPMS, sometimes by using props such as a folded towel, cushion, or chair. Many yoga classes end with meditation, which helps the mind relax. *Tai chi* involves a series of movements in slow motion. Like yoga, it is noncompetitive and encourages a meditative mental state. *The Pilates* exercise system offers many of the same benefits as yoga. These are discussed in greater detail in Chapter 7.

Stress

Many stressful situations are common with MS, some of which also play a role in depression and anxiety, including:

- ▶ Uncertainty (while waiting for a definite diagnosis)
- ▶ The development of new symptoms
- ▶ The need to adjust and readjust to changing abilities

▶ Financial stress and concerns about employment

▶ The presence or possibility of cognitive impairment

▶ Loss of control over some aspects of daily living

▶ Family-related stress

▶ The need to make decisions about new treatments and adjust to those that you choose

Does stress make MS symptoms worse? Many people with MS experience more symptoms during stressful times, and their symptoms seem less troubling or severe when stress abates. This makes sense, because more energy is needed to think, solve problems, and handle daily life during times of stress. Symptoms may be experienced more strongly because the energy we need to deal with them and get on with our lives has been drained.

There is no "right" way to cope with stress. Even within a family, some members might want to talk about MS, read about it, and participate in support groups, while others may ignore it much of the time.

Begin to deal with stress by identifying its sources, which may include:

▶ **Social stressors:** Strong feelings based on interactions with other people. For example, you can be stressed when giving a speech, meeting someone new, or expressing anger.

▶ **Work stressors:** Pressures or tensions related to your job, volunteer work, or homemaking role. For example, you can be stressed when asking the boss for break time during the day, dealing with deadlines, or supervising new employees.

▶ **Mental stressors:** Fears and anxieties, such as worrying about bills or finances, taking an exam, or dealing with family problems.

▶ **Physical stressors:** Strains on our bodies from aches or pains, using heavy equipment, or not sleeping enough.

▶ **Environmental stressors:** Aspects of our surroundings, including noisy offices or restaurants, exhaust fumes, or cold or hot weather.

Here are some ideas that many people find useful to relieve or reduce stress, and feel more relaxed:

▶ **Physical:** As with depression and anxiety, any regular physical activity or fitness program will reduce stress and improve your physical and mental health. Exercise has a relaxing effect; it helps with falling asleep, and reduces high blood pressure. Combine exercise with better nutrition. Having a balanced, healthy diet will pay huge dividends in overall wellness and lowered stress.

▶ **Emotional:** Mental health professionals, including psychologists, psychiatrists, social workers, occupational therapists, and pastoral counselors, can help you identify the sources of your stress and learn to deal with them.

▶ **Spiritual:** Achieving balance in your life will help you feel centered and better able to cope and reduce stress.

Addressing spiritual issues will help you reduce stress by achieving feelings of empowerment, being true to yourself, and becoming connected and involved. Activities such as yoga, meditation, prayer, contemplation, visualization, and relaxation can all be helpful.

▶ **Intellectual:** Addressing cognitive issues will help relieve the stress associated with them. Regain your sense of control by learning more about the disease and developing specific strategies to deal with it. Learning something new will also help keep your mind sharp.

▶ **Social:** Living with MS constantly challenges your social skills. If you are limited in your ability to get around, use e-mail and the Internet to communicate with friends and

Spiritual fitness is a concept of constantly reidentifying myself. Using a wheelchair, I'm redefining myself. Using the walker, redefining myself. Spiritual fitness means constantly reidentifying myself in positive ways, taking negative circumstances and channeling them into positive outcomes. It's a very hard thing to do sometimes.

— Tom

relatives, as well as to obtain information of all kinds. Build recreation and travel into your life; see the resources in Appendix 2.

Cognitive Changes

The term *cognition* refers to brain functions that include comprehension and speech fluency, attention and information processing, memory, and "executive" functions such as planning and problem-solving.

Major cognitive changes are less common in PPMS than in relapsing remitting MS (RRMS), as PPMS is largely a spinal cord disease, but it does occur in a significant number of people. These changes can affect a range of functions, including attention, memory, speed of processing information, problem solving, conceptual reasoning, and learning new information.

Once the problem is identified, it is often a source of relief to people who might have misinterpreted its effects. For example, family members who thought a person with PPMS wasn't paying attention to family matters, or didn't care, are often relieved to learn that the behavior has a basis in PPMS. They can then make adjustments to minimize at least some of the problems.

Compensatory strategies include writing things down or keeping notes using a handheld organizer. Establishing routines can help you overcome problems with memory and judgment. An occupational therapist (OT) or a speech and language pathologist can help you develop strategies for safety and repetition, and written cues can help embed them into your memory.

SEEK AN "MS FREE ZONE"

Dr. Rosalind Kalb refers to an "MS-free zone" as a place where the disease cannot reach. For one person, this might be reading, listening to music, or using a computer. For another, it might be involvement in religious activities or volunteering. Look inside yourself to discover what activities provide emotional respite from PPMS and its day-to-day challenges, so that you can reenergize and refuel your emotional reserves.

Family and Social Issues

As primary progressive multiple sclerosis (PPMS) progresses, it affects everyone in the family. The loss of some abilities, and the inability or difficulty with participating in once taken-for-granted activities, can produce fundamental changes in traditional life roles. Most often, a spouse finds that she or he needs to take on roles that were once the domain of the person with PPMS. This can be stressful for everyone involved.

Family roles can be turned upside down, and people who are unprepared for caregiving may find themselves thrust into new positions of responsibility. A spouse may suddenly feel more like a parent than a partner. At times, family members try to do so much that it discourages the person with PPMS from coping independently. Each family member has his or her own individual emotions, and their feelings will often be out of sync with each other. One might be overwhelmed with anger, while another might be cushioned in calm denial. Even in loving families, it is easy for communication to break down.

The strategy advocated by Dr. Rosalind Kalb in *Multiple Sclerosis: A Guide for Families* is to treat MS as an "uninvited guest" that must not be given more room in the household than it absolutely needs. Families need to seek a reasonable balance between the demands that PPMS places on their resources—financial, emotional, and social—and the needs of all family members.

This is easier said than done, and it requires ongoing communication among family members, especially when family roles change with new symptoms or an increasing level of PPMS-related disability. Chapters of the National MS Society and the MS Association of America have information and resources that may be helpful, and they will make referrals to qualified professionals who can help you with these types of problems.

I gave up cooking when my daughter was 9, and she was about 10 when I stopped driving. Dave was doing my jobs and his job, and I felt horrible for him.
— Shelley

Families cope with the diagnosis of PPMS in various ways. Some handle their issues at family meetings, where everyone is allowed his or her say; others do better talking to each other one-on-one, perhaps in a neutral place away from the home. Mental health professionals can be extremely helpful, because they are trained to help people work through their feelings about MS and talk more openly about difficult subjects. Spiritual advisors also might be important resources.

Those families that seem to cope most effectively develop a *carepartnership*, in which they find ways to meet each others needs, collaborate on planning and decision-making, and share the challenges of dealing with the disease.

Having a healthy relationship is hard work even in the best of times. PPMS can make it even harder. Contact your local National MS Society chapter to learn about the *Relationship Matters* program, which was developed to help couples minimize the impact of MS on their lives.

How Can PPMS Affect a Couple's Relationships?

Intimacy involves all the ways that partners connect with each other. It rests on a foundation of trust, communication, shared goals and expectations, and mutual respect and concern. PPMS can affect intimacy in many ways. Although these changes might at times feel overwhelming, there are satisfying ways to deal with them.

Although sexual difficulties often occur as the direct result of PPMS, they are often not the most important cause of intimacy issues. However, the biggest challenge to a couple's intimacy comes from unexpressed feelings, mood changes, and the emotional and attitudinal changes that often accompany role shifts within their established relationship. A number of spouses in the PPMS focus groups discussed how difficult it is for them to feel sexual attraction toward a person who functions in a very different role in their partnership than was previously the case, or who requires regular hands-on care. Fatigue, experienced by both the person with PPMS and the carepartner, may contribute to the feeling that romance is the last thing on anyone's mind.

> *The most important thing was that we had a strong marriage before the MS, and we had good communication skills. We got help when we hit an impasse, when we had an argument that we couldn't work out. — Shelley*

Cognitive issues present a special set of problems (see Chapter 8). For example, family members might perceive the person with PPMS as uncaring, insensitive, or unconcerned because they have trouble remembering things that are important to others. Recognizing these issues, and addressing them whenever possible, can make a major difference in family dynamics.

SEXUAL CHANGES ASSOCIATED WITH PPMS

People bring their values and personal histories with them when they develop PPMS, and adapting to changes in the area of sexuality might be more difficult than dealing with changes in other aspects of daily living.

Sexual dysfunction is a common problem in PPMS. For example, many men note some form of erectile dysfunction, and women may experience decreased sensation or numbness in the vaginal area. Both can experience decreased libido and interest in sexual activity.

As discussed earlier, PPMS produces symptoms that are referred to as primary, secondary, and tertiary, and sexual dysfunction can be the result of problems at any of these levels. Lesions in the nervous system produce primary symptoms that can reduce sexual drive and genital sensation, arousal, muscle tone, and orgasm. Secondary problems affecting sexual activity can arise from other MS symptoms—such as fatigue, spasticity, or bladder issues—as well as from some of the medications used to treat symptoms. Other problems, such as performance anxiety or changes in family roles, also can affect sexual feelings and performance.

Many sexual problems associated with PPMS *can* be managed successfully. A good first step is to learn to talk about issues of sex and intimacy with your partner, but this is not always an easy thing to do. If symptoms interfere with sexual activity, discuss them with your physician or nurse.

A psychologist or other counselor can help, especially if the person with PPMS has an advanced level of disability, and caregiving needs affect the balance in the couple's partnership. It is very important that both partners be involved in all counseling and discussions. Counseling can be especially helpful in supporting your efforts to deal with painful feelings. It can also teach you how to communicate more effectively with family members and friends, and think through problems to find solutions.

One helpful step is to contact your local National MS Society chapter to learn about the *Relationship Matters* program, which was developed to help couples minimize the impact of MS on their lives, as well as the *Intimacy: Enriching Your Relationship* course. These and other programs and materials from the National MS Society and the MS Association of America are listed in the Resources section.

Please consider these suggestions:

▶ Work at sharing feelings honestly with your partner, so that relatively minor problems don't become major ones.

▶ There are virtually limitless variations of sexual technique and expression. A bit of imagination and ingenuity will go a long way in helping you deal with the physical changes caused by PPMS.

▶ Physical symptoms can interfere with sexual pleasure, and treating them appropriately can make a significant difference. For example, medications to reduce muscle spasms and stiffness can often be timed so they don't interfere with sexual activity.

▶ Many people with PPMS experience reduced genital sensation. Many parts of the body are sensitive to touch, and a bit of patience and skill can result in enhanced pleasure.

▶ Whenever possible, avoid taking sedatives or antidepressant medications before having sex; although antianxiety medications can be helpful in some cases. If you take any of these medications, discuss their dosage and timing with your physician or nurse.

▶ Physical exhaustion, lack of sleep, emotional turmoil, too much heat, overeating, or excess alcohol can interfere with *anyone's* sexual enjoyment. A bit of planning can make sure that these factors do not adversely affect your relationship.

▶ If you are sensitive to heat, a tepid-to-cool bath may improve sexual performance, just as it improves other physical functions.

▶ Painful sensations, such as sharp or burning pain and tingling, may be relieved with ice packs (frozen peas work very well).

▶ Many men, with or without PPMS, experience erectile dysfunction—the inability to produce a firm erection. There are many ways to manage this problem, including drugs such as Viagra®, Cialis®, and Levitra®, as well as injections, and pumps. Your physician or nurse can help you choose the method most appropriate for you.

▶ Always empty your bladder just before sex. If you experience a bit of leakage, remember that urine is sterile and no real damage is done.

HOW DOES PPMS AFFECT YOUR CHILDREN?

Children in families with MS can feel anger, frustration, and grief, just as their parents and adult family members do. They may experience guilt and be concerned that something they did caused their parent to become sick. They may also feel neglected as a result of the focus on the needs of the parent with PPMS.

> My children were 3 and 5, and obviously they could only absorb a certain amount of this. But they could understand that Mom was sick, that Mom was tired a lot, that she couldn't do some of the things that other moms did.
>
> — Shelley

You can be a good parent even if you have substantial disability. You might not be able to throw a softball, but you *can* be a good listener, advocate, and loving presence, spending quality time with your child. Listening, acknowledging a child's feelings, and providing encouragement can meet your child's emotional needs.

Depending on their age, children can usually understand that a parent cannot control the physical symptoms that sometimes interfere with family activities or make it impossible for a parent to be as supportive as everyone would like. They may have more difficulty understanding invisible symptoms such as fatigue, especially since their own energy is almost boundless. Cognitive issues can present a special problem. They not only can be misinterpreted—as not really caring, for example—but they can interfere with family plans and commitments.

> I don't think our kids have been damaged by the MS. They had a lot more responsibility than many of their friends, and they knew how to handle it. As adults, these behaviors have stood them well in their jobs and family life.
>
> — Shelley

Contact the National MS Society to learn about the *Keep S'myelin* newsletter, a fun and engaging resource designed to help children and their parents talk and learn about MS together. Each issue contains stories, interviews, games, and activities that highlight specific topics related to MS, as well as a section just for parents.

Be sure to keep the lines of communication open. If you don't tell your children what is happening, their imaginations will take over—and their imaginations have no limits! They will feel more secure if you provide them with information directly, and they are allowed to ask any questions that might be troubling them. Kids might have difficulty coming to terms with a parent's disability, but they will also learn valuable life skills from an inspiring parent with MS.

Our 5-year-old asked if Shelley was going to die, and we said no, she wouldn't die but she could have different symptoms. They pretty much accepted that.

— Dave

CAN I HAVE (MORE) CHILDREN?

Deciding to have a child is always a serious matter, with or without a partner's PPMS. There is no one right decision, only the one that is right for you and your family. Women with MS do not tend to have more difficulty during pregnancy, and those with relapsing remitting MS (RRMS) actually tend to have fewer attacks. Specific data on women with PPMS are not available.

No matter which spouse has PPMS, you need to think about the effects that increasing physical symptoms, fatigue, and possible cognitive problems might have on the family unit. The most important issue when deciding whether to have children includes the ability to provide emotional support, consistent structure to their lives, and a value system that prepares them for adult life. Children bring joy to our lives, and many people with PPMS make the decision to have children, or additional children, in that light. Others might decide differently.

RELATIONSHIPS WITH FRIENDS

There are often two groups of people in our lives—individuals who are very important to us, and those we consider acquaintances. Some

Shelley has been extremely effective at keeping her network of friends, and they've always been amazingly helpful. She learned a long time ago that you've got to ask your friends for help, and you can't be just embarrassed to say, "Oh, I can't do this, can you help us out?" — Dave

acquaintances might drop out of your life if it becomes more complicated to do things together. But if you can focus on the people most important to you, they are likely to remain good friends and be supportive. Some can become even closer with time.

Because many people do not understand MS, they may make assumptions about what you can or cannot do, based on how they perceive your level of disability. It's helpful to gain comfort and skill in knowing how to handle situations such as:

▶ How to ask for help when you need it
▶ Declining unwanted help
▶ Facilitating communication
▶ Disclosing nonvisible disabilities (such as fatigue or sensory loss)
▶ Dealing with reactions to assistive equipment (such as a cane or wheelchair)
▶ Managing bowel and bladder problems when out in the community
▶ Handling unwanted questions
▶ Acknowledging any disability

REMAINING PRODUCTIVE IF YOU ARE NO LONGER WORKING

If you need to leave work because PPMS symptoms make it difficult to continue working, consider finding other activities that are personally rewarding and that enhance your feelings of self-worth. Don't make decisions too quickly—explore your many options and consider "trying out" activities that you think might work for you.

You also need to consider all aspects of your physical and emotional health. If you don't have an exercise routine, now is the time to start one; a physical therapist can help you with this. Keep your family and friends close, and look to expand your social support network by exploring what your community has to offer. Consider taking time to develop interests you might not previously have had time for; volunteering may become a viable option that you didn't have time for previously.

I'd always been very independent and I enjoyed what I did from a work standpoint. How was not working going to redefine my life? It would be a pretty big change. — Kathy

LEISURE ACTIVITIES

There is no need to abandon leisure activity because of MS. You can still enjoy most of the activities you did before the diagnosis, even if they need to be modified to accommodate fatigue or mobility issues. Everything from yoga to bowling or skiing can be modified. Many areas have developed adaptive recreation programs. Check with your local National MS Society chapter or the MS Association of America, the recreation council in your community, or the Chamber of Commerce of your city or one you plan to visit. If your city has limited access to its public institutions or transportation system, become an advocate for change.

Listen to your body and kind of know what your body is capable of doing, and then find ways that you can still do the things that you enjoy doing.
— Kathy

E-MAIL AND THE INTERNET

E-mail and the Internet have become the preferred way for many people to communicate with friends and relatives, as well as being a great source of information of all kinds. This can be very beneficial to people with PPMS, especially if you have problems with mobility or symptoms such as fatigue.

There is also a lot of really great information on the Internet, but you need to filter out what you're looking for. I usually go to the National MS Society's site.

— Jason

A good way to get started is to evaluate your interests, needs, and resources to determine how to take advantage of what the computer and Internet offer. You also need to assess your workstation comfort and design, so you will stay healthy while you "surf the information highway."

Many people use the computer and Internet to:

▶ Keep in touch with friends and family without leaving home
▶ Keep a record of finances
▶ Pay bills
▶ Order groceries and have them delivered
▶ Play games
▶ Talk online in a chat room with others who have MS
▶ Access the latest information about MS
▶ Write stories or letters
▶ Help yourself and your family with school projects

The MS Association of America offers an online Networking Program for individuals with MS, as well as carepartners, to exchange e-mail for support, information, and friendship.

TRAVEL

A number of sources are available to help with issues relating to travel. For example, all airlines, bus companies, and Amtrak offer special assistance to passengers, and the national parks provide special information for visitors with disabilities. Most major hotel chains, and many independent ones, have adapted rooms to meet your special needs.

Carepartner Support and Resources*

Primary progressive multiple sclerosis (PPMS) is associated with a higher incidence of disability than other forms of MS. This must be considered when planning for the future. The best motto is "hope for the best, plan for the worst." This chapter is written for carepartners and family members, but it will be useful for readers who have PPMS as well, because it will give you a better understanding of the stress that your carepartner and family is experiencing.

Help and support are available from many sources. A good place to start is with *Caring for Loved Ones with Advanced MS: A Guide for Families*, a National MS Society publication, and through the MS Association of America's Helpline.

When a family member—most often a spouse—becomes a carepartner because of advanced MS, many areas of family life can be affected, including:

▶ **Loss of income because of carepartner duties and changes in family roles:** In addition to the person with PPMS, carepartners

---

*In this chapter, we use the terms *carepartner* and *caregiver* interchangeably. However, this terminology is in flux among professionals, who are moving toward using the terms *primary carepartner* for spouses and other family members who provide care, *carepartner* for anyone—paid or unpaid—who provides care, but the term *caregiver* remains in common usage.

may have reduced or lost income because more time is required at home. This can cause a significant financial burden.

▶ **Loss of time to care for your own needs:** Family carepartners often neglect taking care of themselves.

▶ **Changes in your partnership with your loved one:** Intimacy can fade in many ways, from companionship and conversation to the loss of sexual intimacy. It becomes increasingly important to find joy in the small things of life, and to spend time nurturing the things that both of you care about.

The most critical issues facing family members who become care-partners are emotional and stress-related. As described by Drs. Deborah Miller and Peggy Crawford, one important key to maintaining the health of your relationship is to consider each other as *carepartners* rather than care-giver and care-receiver. Emphasizing the responsibility that partners have to each other will help put the situation in better perspective and allow you to maintain the bonds of partnership with less strain. It is criti-cal that the partner with PPMS be respectful, caring, and appreciative of the efforts of the carepartner, and that there is mutual respect and caring.

Carepartner issues that can arise include:

▶ Caring for a physically-challenged loved one can be physically and emotionally exhausting, and carepartners are at increased risk for depression and anxiety.

▶ Analysis of the North American Research Committee on MS (NARCOMS) data showed that about half the carepartners had missed work during the previous year because of caregiving responsibilities, and 7 percent had been forced to make changes in their jobs as a result of these responsibilities.

▶ Stress places carepartners at higher risk for a variety of illnesses, because they tend to neglect their own health and wellness. It is critical that carepartners attend to their own health needs, includ-ing regular medical checkups, exercise, and good nutrition.

- Primary carepartners need time to pursue their individual interests.
- Carepartners often feel guilty about doing anything for themselves. We recommend the well-spouse programs sponsored by the National Association of Home Care (NAHC) and the other programs for caregivers and carepartners listed in Appendix 2.

CAREPARTNER STRAIN AND BURDEN

Carepartner strain—often referred to as *burnout*—may be thought of as a state of physical, emotional, and mental exhaustion that results from long-term caregiving responsibility and the stress associated with having a partner with a chronic medical condition, often with insufficient respite. If you are a caregiver or carepartner, support is available. This might include getting assistance with home care, reducing isolation, restoring balance to your life, receiving respite care, and generally avoiding becoming overwhelmed by being forced to take on too many roles.

> *One of the things I try to do is develop some activities that don't involve Shelley, because we're together an awful lot. We do a lot of things together socially, and I think it's healthy to have a few activities that get me away.*
> — Dave

What Are the Signs of Carepartner Stress That Can Lead to Burnout?

Emotional signs of stress include chronic irritability or resentment, feeling down in the dumps, continual boredom, excessive nervousness/anxiety, feeling overwhelmed, and nightmares. *Thought-related signs* of stress include constant worrying, distractibility, expecting the worst to happen, and difficulty making everyday decisions. *Physical signs* include clammy hands or sweating, constipation/diarrhea, dry mouth, headache, heart palpitations, stomachaches, nausea, muscle

I don't want Dave to just feel that he can't do things like going fishing. I want him to be able to do those things. He's done a couple of short trips, and girlfriends come over to stay, and we have a pajama party. So everybody is happy to be in a new environment. I don't want him to have to feel that "I can't go because of Shelley." That would make me feel terrible. I want him to go, and I want him to have a good time. — Shelley

spasms or tightness, a lump in the throat, faintness, fatigue/weariness, sleeping too much or too little, and short or shallow breathing.

When you feel overwhelmed with stress, sharing problems with others can help relieve your feelings and give you a new perspective. All National MS Society chapters have affiliated self-help groups, and many have groups and programs for caregivers. Several national caregiver organizations provide materials specifically addressing caregiver stress, including the National Family Caregivers Association and the Well-Spouse Foundation.

Respite Care Resources

Contact your county and/or state Department of Human Services, or your local Office on Aging, to find out what programs are available for family caregivers. Some states have found that funding for respite care helps avoid more expensive nursing home stays. Although historically many of these programs have focused on elderly carepartners, an increasing number are now providing services more generally. These programs can also be a way to access homemaker services, personal attendant services, meal delivery, and case management services. Other options include:

▶ Explore nonprofit organizations and faith-based groups that offer respite services. For example, Faith-in-Action is a nationwide network of volunteers who provide nonmedical help and respite for people with long-term care needs.

▶ Check with the National MS Society or the MS Association of America to learn about available services in your community.

TWELVE STEPS FOR CAREPARTNERS

1. Although I cannot control the disease process, I need to remember I can control many aspects of how it affects me and my loved one.

2. I need to take care of myself, so that I can continue doing the things that are most important.

3. I need to simplify my lifestyle, so that my time and energy are available for things that are really important at this time.

4. I need to cultivate the gift of allowing others to help me, because caring for my loved one is too big a job to be done by one person.

5. I need to take one day at a time rather than worry about what might or might not happen in the future.

6. I need to structure my day because a consistent schedule makes life easier.

7. I need to have a sense of humor because laughter helps to put things in a more positive perspective.

8. I need to remember that my loved one is not being difficult on purpose; rather the behavior and emotions are being distorted by the illness.

9. I need to focus on and enjoy what my loved one can still do rather than constantly lament over what is gone.

10. I need to increasingly depend upon other relationships for additional love and support.

11. I need to frequently remind myself that I am doing the best that I can at this very moment.

12. I need to seek out spiritual support and nourish my spiritual life.

Permission to reprint this list was granted by Carol J. Farran, D.N.Sc, R.N.; and Eleanora Keene-Haggerty, M.A. It is based on the Alcoholics Anonymous Twelve-Step Program, for caregivers of people with dementia.

▶ Visit www.lotsahelpinghands.com, a national caregiver coordination service that allows family, friends, neighbors, and colleagues to more easily assist with daily meals, rides, shopping, babysitting, errands, etc.

▶ Check the website of the Family Caregiver Alliance (www.caregiver.org) for a state-by-state listing of respite and other services for family carepartners.

▶ Explore adult day programs in your community that provide respite to carepartners.

▶ Learn about nursing homes that set aside beds for respite.

▶ Identify Veterans Affairs (VA) hospitals that offer respite for families of veterans.

▶ Finally, if you have no other alternative, and can manage it, hire and pay someone to provide in-home respite care. Remember, family members who cannot provide hands-on assistance might be willing to assist with paid services. Ask yourself:

  • Do I need regular or occasional help?

  • What times would be best?

  • How much advance notice does the substitute care provider need?

WHEN FAMILY CARE IS NOT ENOUGH

Advanced PPMS can lead to a level of disability that requires a higher level of care than family members are able to provide. Planning ahead will make this easier. The best time to become an "educated consumer" is not when you are in the midst of a crisis, but earlier, when you can take your time to learn about options and gather information for possible future reference. The following is an overview of available resources and services.

Home Care Services

One of the greatest fears of people facing advanced disease is that they will have to enter a nursing home facility, separated from family and surrounded by frail and elderly people. Home- and community-based services can help people remain in their homes as long as possible and provide services and interventions that enhance independence. They are often more flexible than institutional care facilities in meeting an individual's needs.

Community-Based Home Care Services

Many community services are available to help people with a chronic disease or disability to remain in their homes. By offering support, nursing care, rehabilitation, and medication management, home-based services can decrease hospital admissions and avoid premature and expensive nursing home placement. They include:

▶ **Certified nursing assistants (CNAs) or home health aides:** Assist with daily living tasks under medical supervision, usually by a visiting nurse.

▶ **Personal care attendants or personal care assistants:** Help with activities of daily living (ADLs), such as dressing, bathing, toileting, transferring, and eating.

▶ **Visiting nurses:** Provide assistance with medications, catheter care, wound care, and similar matters.

▶ **Housekeepers:** Provide basic homemaking tasks, light cleaning, errands, laundry, and cooking.

▶ **Rehabilitation specialists:** Including occupational, physical, and speech therapists, who provide a wide range of services that promote independence and make it easier to deal with the symptoms of PPMS.

Check with the National MS Society, the MS Association of America, the Well Spouse Association, the National Family Caregivers Association, or a local Center for Independent Living to learn what is available in your community.

You first need to think about what services you need—what kind of help, how much help, and when you need it. The level of skill for each service varies, as does the cost:

- ▶ **Skilled care paid for by Medicare:** If a physician orders "skilled care" provided by a registered nurse or physical therapist, Medicare or insurance companies might cover the cost. This care is usually provided on an intermittent or short-term basis. An assessment by a nurse or therapist will probably be required to document the need for skilled care. Home health care organizations that provide skilled care will bill Medicare directly; they will discuss what is covered with the family.

- ▶ **Home care paid by insurance or Medicare:** Many long-term care insurance policies provide for home health care or personal care services, but they have specific policies whose rules must be met. Medicaid usually covers some home health care services. You might wish to consult with a social service worker for more information and to discuss financial eligibility.

- ▶ **Additional services provided by an agency:** Many home health agencies, registries, and referral services can provide nurses, home health aides, and companions on an hourly basis. Most agencies require a minimum of 4 hours of care, and some provide live-in assistance.

It is helpful to clarify whether you will hire an agency or hire an individual directly. This decision will be determined by your financial resources and/or health insurance coverage, as well as by any government benefits for which you are eligible. You will need to decide who will interview the applicants, where they will be interviewed, and who will oversee paying them. If you hire directly, you will probably need to have someone (such as an accountant) to help with the financial responsibilities of being an employer in terms of taxes, insurance, and related matters. It is important to conduct a background check, and review both personal and professional references. If the person will live with you, consider privacy issues for both you and your employee. See Appendix 2 for more specific information.

Adult Day Care

Adult day care programs can help people live in their community when they need more services than can be provided at home. These services also offer an opportunity to socialize in a protected environment. Although many programs are geared toward the elderly, some have a mixed-age clientele, and others are geared specifically to MS. You can obtain information about programs in your area through the National MS Society, the MS Association of America, and the National Adult Day Services Association. Some of the expense may be covered by insurance, Medicare, or Medicaid.

ASSISTED LIVING

We usually think of assisted living as designed for the elderly, but younger people with disabilities increasingly use this type of housing. The Assisted Living Federation of America, the National Center for Assisted Living, and your local MS organizations can provide information about options in your area.

NURSING HOME CARE

If PPMS progresses to the point at which 24-hour skilled nursing care is essential, the needs of the person with PPMS can exceed family resources. Significant cognitive loss, incontinence, nutritional compromise, and/or respiratory issues require complex clinical care. If the family is no longer able to carry out these responsibilities, even with additional assistance at home, a nursing home might be the best option for everyone.

This does not mean you will be less involved in each other's lives. Many families find that their relationships improve when all of their energy is not spent meeting daily care needs. You can visit the nursing home frequently, sometimes to help with tasks like eating, but often just to visit and be together. Family members can return to their former roles. If you feel less stress, your time together will probably be less stressful as well. Remember that many nursing home residents return home for holidays and special visits. There are many ways you can continue to be closely involved.

In addition, people with PPMS may find that socialization opportunities and programs make a facility desirable and enjoyable, especially given the growing trend of separating younger people into a "neighborhood" in which their special needs can be addressed.

11

Economic Issues

Everyone needs to plan for the future. This is particularly important for people with primary progressive multiple sclerosis (PPMS) and their families, because the disease is often associated with a high degree of disability and unemployment.

This chapter is a general introduction to the economic issues associated with PPMS. Appendix 2 can direct you to many excellent and detailed resources.

EMPLOYMENT

Depending on your symptoms, health issues, and degree of disability, you may need to deal with situations that temporarily or permanently affect your ability to work, or that slow down your natural path of career development.

Although 90 percent of people with MS have a history of employment, in the Slifka study approximately 62 percent were employed 5 years after diagnosis; this percentage was about the same for people with PPMS and relapsing remitting MS (RRMS). However, with time, the differences widen; only 18 percent of those with PPMS were still working 12 years after diagnosis, as compared to 58 percent of those with RRMS.

It is essential that you address any barriers to continuing work as early as possible, but not so quickly that you have not considered a variety of alternatives. Consider these suggestions:

I was painfully aware that others, and specifically people who could control my destiny, were probably very aware that I was really struggling just to do simple things. And they didn't know why. When I finally decided to disclose, I talked to the vice president of human resources, and I'm very glad that I did. He handled that information very confidentially, and talked with me about whether or not there were things I needed in the workplace.

— Kathy

▶ Review your work situation as it relates to your symptoms. Some types of work are affected by PPMS more quickly or directly than others. For example, if you experience fatigue or weakness, you will be much more affected if you work in a production line setting than if you work in an office.

▶ Make sure that you are familiar with the benefits to which you are entitled. All employees in a group plan must be given the same health benefits, regardless of health status. The Health Insurance Portability and Accountability Act (HIPPA) allows you to change jobs and go from one group plan to another without any limitations on preexisting conditions, provided this is done no more than once a year, and that you have had at least one year of coverage in a previous position.

▶ If your work schedule is a problem, consider switching to part-time. Before you make any decisions, find out whether your benefits will be reduced. A viable alternative might be to discuss a more flexible work schedule with your employer.

▶ You have more rights and protections when you are employed. Even if MS symptoms are interfering with your job performance, explore all possible alternatives before leaving your job. Only after you determine that reasonable adaptations have failed should you explore other options, such as retraining, finding another job, working less, or stopping work. You are protected by the Americans with Disabilities Act (ADA); check the U.S. Department of Labor website at www.dol.gov/dol/topic/disability/ada.htm. The laws in Canada are similar.

Disclosure

You have no obligation to disclose your PPMS unless you need accommodations in your workplace or need to take time off because of disability or illness. The decision to disclose is a highly individual matter. There are pros and cons to making your diagnosis public to your employer and coworkers. Disclosure might be helpful if you have visible symptoms or if your symptoms—visible or invisible—interfere with your job performance.

Disclosure will make it easier to discuss with your employer any changes in your workload or pattern that might help you to continue to do the same quality of work as before. Some ways that you can modify your work situation include setting priorities, rearranging your work day so that you take on easier tasks at times when you know your energy will be lower, and arranging your work environment to suit your needs.

Disclosure was a problem because I was working. I didn't know whether I should talk to my supervisor. I was very afraid that I was going to lose my job. Fortunately, I worked in a setting where I did get support. Once I disclosed at least to my supervisors, they were very supportive, and I've been able to move in my career within the system.
— Tom

Don't make this decision without first considering its advantages and disadvantages. Talking about it might lead to positive changes, such as modifications in your workstation. However, it might also lead to problems, such as being moved to a less satisfactory job.

Reasonable Accommodation and Job Retention

Depending on your job responsibilities and MS symptoms, a wide range of adjustments can be made to help you maintain your productivity, for example:

▶ Modifications to your work environment might be helpful, and most are fairly simple and inexpensive. They can include moving your parking spot closer to the office to reduce fatigue; new equipment or changes in access, such as modifications to allow wheelchair access; or moving your workspace to provide more privacy so your thought processes are less likely to be distracted.

▶ Look for ways that your job responsibilities might be modified, or explore whether you might be given a different position that would not involve the same limitations as your present one.

▶ Alter your present work schedule or work at home either part- or full-time.

Vocational Rehabilitation

Vocational rehabilitation services can help you keep your job, return to the work force if you are not working, or help you retrain for a new position. It can be very helpful to contact your state vocational rehabilitation agency when you first begin to have problems in the workplace, rather than wait until a crisis develops. These services can help with vocational assessment, neuropsychological testing to identify memory or related problems, specialty consultations not covered by insurance—including psychotherapy, direct job placements, and assistive technology consultation. See www.nationalmssociety.org/living-with-multiple-sclerosis/employment/index.aspx for helpful suggestions.

If You Need to Stop Working

If you decide that it is in your best interest to stop working, you will need to consider *Social Security Disability Insurance* (SSDI), the federal insurance program managed by the Social Security Administration. Qualifying for SSDI can be a lengthy process, requiring medical evidence of your inability to work, and you should check with the National MS Society or the MS Association of America if you are considering taking this step. Do not be discouraged if you are denied coverage initially. You should appeal the decision and seek legal assistance if necessary; the chances of getting approved for SSDI are often greater for people who work with an attorney. The National MS Society provides materials for people with MS and their physicians to help with applications for SSDI; visit www.national MSsociety.org/SSDI for more information. The booklet *Social Security Disability Benefits* includes sample letters, and a separate booklet is available for health care professionals with guidelines to help them provide optimal medical information.

When the time came to make the transition not to work totally, there was a lot of fear. What am I going to do with my life? What am I going to do with myself? A lot of my self worth and my significance was tied up in working and being able to accomplish things, and having relationships through work, etc.

— Kathy

LIFE PLANNING AND ADVANCE DIRECTIVES

Life planning is important for everyone. It helps to anticipate what the future might hold and prepare for those possibilities. Planning ahead requires clear communication among family members and discussions about everyone's values and wishes. It also includes thinking about and communicating your wishes and preferences about long-term care and end-of-life issues.

Follow the approach of "plan for the worst and hope for the best." Try to anticipate your possible future needs. Identify the legal documents that everyone involved in your life should have, and take the necessary steps to assure that your wishes and values are reflected in future medical and end-of-life decisions.

What Future Problems Should I Anticipate?

People with PPMS and their families may have to deal with many problems, including physical abilities, independence, financial earning power, emotional ties, and options for the future. Ways that you can improve your future financial health include:

▶ **Maximize your income tax deductions:** You probably already know that you can deduct out-of-pocket medical expenses for doctors, hospitals, emergency room visits, therapies, and other costs if they exceed a certain percentage of your income. However, other costs related to living with a chronic medical condition may also qualify as medical deductions, such as room and board for a personal care assistant, wheelchair repairs, modifications to your home for medical reasons, or wages for personal care services. Consult a qualified tax professional to be sure you are holding on to as much income as possible.

▶ **Maximize your health insurance benefits:** Know what your health plan covers in terms of at-home nursing care, rehabilitation, durable medical equipment, mental health benefits, etc. If your plan offers a disease management or care management program, this could provide additional coordination of care.

▶ **Explore all resources that relate to disability income:** This includes private long-term disability insurance, SSDI, and supplemental security income (SSI) if you have minimal income and resources. Social Security and Veterans Affairs (VA) agencies also provide benefits to family members.

▶ **Investigate Medicaid waiver programs in your state:** Many states focus on keeping people with long-term care needs out of nursing homes and in the community. Although you might not have a low enough income to qualify for standard Medicaid, Medicaid waiver programs provide services to families who have more financial resources than the traditional Medicaid recipient, but who require long-term care services.

▶ **Consult with a certified financial planner and/or an elder law attorney:** Make sure you are optimally managing your finances and protecting your assets.

What Legal Documents Should I Have?

Everyone should have the basic documents in place that allow a trusted relative or friend to make health care decisions on their behalf, should the time come when they are unable to make them for themselves. Make sure that enough information has been shared so that any decisions that need to be made will accurately reflect your wishes.

It's been very important to realize that some time in the future—how far and how fast I don't know—I am going to be worse off than I am right now. To know that in advance is very, very important, because it allows me to prepare ahead of time.
— Tom

Your Will

You and your loved ones should have current wills drawn up by an attorney, and they should be kept up-to-date. If you do not have a will, the laws of the state where you live will dictate where your property goes and who will administer your estate. Wills also provide an opportunity for your wishes to be stated with regard to guardianship of minor children and management of their assets until they are old enough to assume direct control.

Advance Directives

The term *advance directive* refers to those documents that allow people to achieve control over their health care, should they become unable to make decisions for themselves. They are most often done when wills are prepared. Advance directive requirements vary greatly among states and should be drawn up in consultation with an attorney who is familiar with the laws of your state. The most common directives are:

▶ **Living will:** Also referred to as an *advance medical directive.* This document spells out your wishes about medical care should you become unable to state those wishes. It says what you want to happen in specific medical situations, such as the placement of a feeding tube or the use of mechanical ventilation. Many states only allow a living will to be utilized when a person is terminally ill, in a coma, or in a persistent vegetative state.

▶ **Health care proxy:** Also referred to as a *medical power of attorney,* this directive allows you to name a personal representative to make medical decisions on your behalf should your decision-making become impaired. It is critical that your designated representative understand your values, beliefs, and desires, and that any decision he or she makes reflects your wishes as outlined in your living will.

▶ **Do Not Resuscitate (DNR) Order:** This document instructs medical personnel not to use cardiopulmonary resuscitation (CPR) if your heart stops beating. Some states have a variation of this directive specifically for Emergency Medical Services personnel.

It is important to review these documents regularly, and to draft new ones if your wishes change. As long as a person is mentally able, these directives can be revoked at any time. Remember, if *you* do not choose a person to make medical decisions when you are unable to do so, a court will appoint someone to make them.

Special Needs Trusts

People who are under 65 and disabled can establish a special needs trust that allows them to *shelter* assets. This allows them to keep their assets and also be eligible for government benefits such as SSI, Medicaid, or housing vouchers. This type of trust can be particularly useful if you anticipate an inheritance or a personal injury settlement.

Managing Your Financial Resources

We all need to live within our budgets, and this means allocating part of our income to basics such as housing, food, and transportation; part to the pleasures in life such as travel, dinner with friends, and movies; and reserving part of our income for the unexpected. Anyone living with a chronic disease such as PPMS has additional expenses that must also be considered. They include such items as medical costs, including doctor and clinic visits; hospitalizations, prescription and over-the-counter medications, medical supplies, and adaptive equipment; home visits from occupational and physical therapists, nurses, and others; and home and vehicle modifications.

In addition to these costs, which are relatively simple to calculate, there are additional economic consequences to living with a progressive disease. They can include "missed opportunity" costs, such as earnings lost as the result of job loss or modification (for example, transitioning to part-time work) or the need for a spouse to limit work hours or leave the work force because of carepartner responsibilities.

This makes the need for financial planning even more important. See Appendix 2 for material that can help you get a handle on this important issue. We especially recommend the booklet *Adapting: Financial Planning for a Life with Multiple Sclerosis*.

Government Benefit Programs

Programs for which established eligibility criteria exist include SSDI, Medicare, Medicaid, and veteran's benefits. Talking with a Social Security Administration benefits counselor is a good way to start; if you are a veteran, organizations such as Paralyzed Veterans of America can help you navigate the process of applying for benefits.

Health Insurance

As we all know, health benefits are a constant concern for many Americans. Canadians and most European do not experience this because they have a universal health care system.

It is essential that you understand the benefits and restrictions of your current health plan and how it can be used to maximally cover your specific needs. Denied and delayed health benefit payments are common. Persistence is time-consuming, but usually worthwhile. Most Americans have health care provided through their employment, which makes the possibility of having to give up working a "double whammy" in terms of its effect on your financial situation!

Become informed about your options ahead of time, so that you can do what is necessary to preserve your health coverage. We refer you to *Health Insurance Resources: A Guide for People with Chronic Disease and Disability*, a comprehensive guide to the insurance maze.

12

How the Multiple Sclerosis Organizations Can Help

People with PPMS and their families have many needs and concerns related to the disease. The issues vary, based on the time since diagnosis, the degree of impairment, and family and work situations. Personality characteristics, previous life events, and learning and coping styles also are involved. Your family physician or neurologist can be a good source of information, but the extensive nonmedical needs of people with PPMS require much more than can be provided by medical specialists. In North America, the primary resources for addressing nonmedical MS-related needs are the National MS Society, the MS Association of America, and the MS Society of Canada. This chapter provides general information about these organizations, as well as specific ways in which they can help you.

THE NATIONAL MULTIPLE SCLEROSIS SOCIETY

733 Third Avenue, New York, NY 10017; 800-FIGHT MS (800-344-4867); www.nationalmssociety.org

The Society's mission is to mobilize people and resources to drive research for a cure and to address the challenges of everyone affected by MS. It helps people affected by MS by funding cutting-edge research, promoting change through advocacy, facilitating professional education, and providing programs and services that help people with MS and their families move their lives forward. The Society is the largest nonprofit organization in the United States that supports national and international research on the prevention, cure, and treatment of MS. To date, it has expended more than $500 million in research funding.

The Society has more than 500,000 members, including more than 360,000 people who have MS. A 50-state network of chapters provides assistance and education for those living with the disease. Home offices in New York City, Denver, and Washington, D.C. direct MS-related research and advocacy, provide some specific services, and provide support, structure, and guidance for local chapters. The Society's national Information Resource Center is staffed by highly trained human service professionals who respond to nearly 20,000 inquiries every month. This call center is the entry point into the *MS Navigator* program, which ensures that anyone with an MS-related need will receive timely, customized help to find resources and solutions.

All Society chapters offer financial assistance for certain goods and services when community resources fall short, and most also offer care management services for the complex situations that people with PPMS might encounter. In addition, the Society offers multiple ways for people living with MS to connect with each other, including a network of more than 1,700 self-help groups and trained peer support volunteers. Professional education initiatives and a system of affiliated MS centers promote access to quality health care.

A National Board of Directors, composed of business and professional leaders with a special interest in MS, establishes society policies and priorities. The Board is assisted by a nationally representative group of individuals with MS, the National Programs Advisory Council. A Board of Trustees governs each local chapter. Staff at both national and chapter levels work in partnership with volunteers and the community to implement the necessary and desired programs. An ongoing process of identifying needs and eliciting feedback regarding the value of programs involves people with MS, their families, and the professionals who serve them, and provides direction for Society activities.

Philosophy of National MS Society Programs

The Society is committed to expanding knowledge of MS, enhancing access to MS specialty medical care, and empowering people with MS to live as independently as possible within the limits of their disabilities and to the maximum of their capabilities within the least restrictive environment. These goals are achieved through national and local programs and activities that lead to the implementation or continuation of one or more of the *Principles to Promote Quality of Life for People with MS* developed by the MS International Federation (MSIF).

Society programs and services are designed to:

- ▶ Inform and educate people with MS and their families, professionals, public officials, and the general public about MS
- ▶ Provide support programs and services that help people with MS and their families cope with the changes and challenges of MS
- ▶ Help people gain access to community resources and quality, specialty health care
- ▶ Stimulate changes and developments in the community and public policy beneficial to people affected by MS
- ▶ Fill gaps in community resources
- ▶ Provide direct service to address critical needs, including financial assistance for certain goods and services when community resources are inadequate

Society services are offered without regard to race, color, religion, age, disability, sexual orientation, or an individual's relationship with a chapter. Chapters do hold "targeted" programs to meet the needs of specific groups, including those who are newly diagnosed, young professionals' groups, and a gay/lesbian network. Initiatives are also being developed to provide programs specifically for people with PPMS.

The confidentiality of members with MS and their family members ("clients") is strictly maintained. Client status is indistinguishable on the general membership list, and clients receive general Society mailings, including solicitations for support, unless a clear request to the contrary is made.

Who Does the National MS Society Serve?

People who have MS are at the center of chapter programs. Since others are affected by the disease as well, Society clients includes everyone who requests information and/or professional assistance. The secondary focus of the Society's programs is the MS "family circle"—spouses, children, parents, other relatives, and significant others. Coworkers and close friends are included in this circle; family members and significant others can also utilize chapter programs.

The Society is the leading source of information about MS for the general public. It also provides education to health professionals, service providers, and community agencies. Although this is not a direct service to people with MS or their families, the information and education provided can significantly impact the quality of life for those affected by MS, through increasing access to quality health care and community resources, and promoting understanding from others.

Quality of Life Principles

The Society embraces the Quality of Life Principles identified by the Multiple Sclerosis International Federation (MSIF) in *The Principles to Promote the Quality of Life of People with MS*. It has adopted these principles as the foundation for its own efforts to address the challenges of each person whose life is affected by MS. They can be summarized as:

- ▶ **Independence and empowerment:** People with MS are empowered as full participants in their communities and in decision-making about the management and treatment of the disease.
- ▶ **Medical care:** People with MS have access to medical care, treatments, and therapies appropriate to their needs.
- ▶ **Continuing (long-term or social) care:** People with MS have access to a wide range of age-appropriate care services that enable them to function as independently as possible.

▶ **Health promotion and disease prevention:** People with MS have the information and services they need to maintain positive health practices and a healthy lifestyle.

▶ **Support for family members:** Family members and caregivers receive information and support to mitigate the effects of MS.

▶ **Transportation:** People with MS have access to their communities through accessible public transportation and assistive technology for personal automobiles.

▶ **Employment and volunteer activities:** Support systems and services are available to enable people with MS to continue employment as long as they are productive and desire to work.

▶ **Disability entitlements and cash assistance:** Disability entitlements and services are available to those in need, provide an adequate standard of living, and have flexibility to allow for the disease variability that is characteristic of multiple sclerosis.

▶ **Education:** MS does not inhibit the education of people with MS, their families, or careers.

▶ **Housing and accessibility of buildings in the community:** Accessibility of public buildings, and the availability of accessible homes and apartments, is essential to independence for people with MS.

MULTIPLE SCLEROSIS ASSOCIATION OF AMERICA

706 Haddonfield Road, Cherry Hill, NJ 08002; 800-532-7667; www.msassociation.org.

The MS Association of America, also known as MSAA, is a national nonprofit organization dedicated to enriching the quality of life for everyone affected by MS. It also promotes greater understanding of the needs and challenges of those who face physical limitations.

Since its founding in 1970, MSAA's philosophy and efforts have focused on programs offering information, support, and assistance to everyone affected by MS. This includes individuals with MS and their family members, carepartners, and friends, as well as medical professionals. A national board of directors oversees its activities and services. These accomplished professionals, some of whom also live with MS, bring their combined experience in medicine, business, and government to MSAA's leadership and governance.

A volunteer Healthcare Advisory Council is comprised of medical professionals who specialize in MS, including neurologists, psychologists, nurses, physical therapists, and occupational therapists. Chaired by MSAA's chief medical officer, this group participates in the design of certain programs and educational materials.

The MS Association of America is staffed by dedicated, compassionate employees and volunteers who strive to help each individual on a personal level. The national office serves clients throughout the United States, and its six regional offices provide assistance on a more local basis, facilitating outreach and awareness.

Offering Lifelines

Individuals with MS, family members, and carepartners can discuss the many issues and emotions that accompany MS with the MS Association of America's experienced, trained, and caring Helpline consultants. They offer information and encouragement, teaming with clients and their carepartners to identify obstacles and discover ways to overcome them. They may also recommend useful programs offered by MSAA that might be of help to the caller. Certain programs, such as equipment distribution and magnetic resonance imaging (MRI) assistance, require clients to submit an application. Helpline consultants can assist callers with the application process. The Helpline also provides a bilingual service to members of the Spanish-speaking community.

The Helpline is an excellent resource for learning about local professionals and services through an extensive national database developed by MSAA's Resource Detectives™ Program. This program employs volunteers to seek out information about programs, professionals, and other local resources.

Helpline consultants can provide information about MS research, treatments, and pharmaceutical assistance programs; legal issues, such as Social Security and Disability Insurance, the Americans with Disabilities Act, and employment; and information about services such as patient education, counseling, rehabilitation, physical and occupational therapy, and wellness programs. They can also help clients and carepartners prepare questions for visits with their physicians.

A Life Coaching program assists individuals with MS to achieve the highest possible level of physical and emotional health. Trained, experienced life coaches lead weekly group sessions by phone or online to teach problem-solving skills using real-life situations. Participants learn strategies that will prove helpful throughout their journey with MS.

Finding Answers

MSAA's publications provide helpful information about a range of subjects, including medical research and treatments, symptom management, health and wellness, complementary and alternative therapies, and coping strategies. Its quarterly magazine, *The Motivator*, contains articles on vital issues, research, treatments, and personal stories.

The MSAA's website is a resource for individuals with MS, families, friends, and anyone interested in learning more about MS and the MS Association of America. The "About Multiple Sclerosis" section features such topics as, "What is MS," "Types of MS," and "Treatments of MS."

Multiple Sclerosis Information (MSi) greatly increases MSAA's ability to serve more clients in more locations through enhanced web technology and updated electronic communications. The MSi educational web video series *A Closer Look* features on-demand programming with experts on MS talking about symptoms, treatments, and disease management and can be viewed at home.

MSAA's free Lending Library offers nearly 300 MS resources on diagnosis, symptoms, treatments, general health, and support, along with books that inspire through personal experiences and life stories. It includes books in Spanish and DVDs of MSi programs and MS-related topics.

Magnetic Resonance Imaging

The MS Association of America provides assistance in obtaining MRI scans, which are used to give doctors the answers they need to help diagnose MS and to get an "inside view" of disease activity.

The MRI Diagnostic Fund helps individuals obtain an initial diagnostic MRI by working with imaging centers and doctors' offices. For individuals with no insurance or who have been denied insurance coverage, MSAA may assist with payment for a diagnostic MRI. To qualify for financial assistance, certain income limits apply.

The MRI Institute provides insurance advocacy and financial assistance to those in need of follow-up MRI exams to examine disease activity and/or treatment effectiveness. Similar to the MRI Diagnostic Fund, certain income limits apply. Individuals with any income level are eligible for advocacy to assist in gaining approval for an MRI through their own insurance companies.

Easing Daily Life

The MS Association of America eases daily life with products and services that increase comfort, safety, and/or mobility. Requested equipment is shipped at no charge. (Certain income requirements apply, as well as limits on the number of items that can be obtained.)

The Equipment Distribution Program provides a variety of equipment at no charge, designed to increase safety and accessibility. This includes bathroom safety items such as tub/shower chairs, grab bars, and raised toilet seats; daily living aids such as reachers and wide-grip utensils; and mobility products that include canes, walkers, and wheelchairs.

The Cooling Equipment Distribution Program helps individuals whose symptoms worsen from heat. In association with the National Aeronautics and Space Administration (NASA), MSAA conducted extensive research into the effects of moderate, controlled cooling on individuals with heat-sensitive MS. The resultant technology enables some people to continue such activities as exercise and physical therapy programs by controlling the effects of heat and reducing fatigue. The program provides cooling apparel kits at no charge. They include a vest, collar, wrist wraps, and a cooling accessory.

MSAA may be able to help people with limited mobility or other physical needs through its Barrier-Free Housing Program. The program offers 125 apartments that are completely wheelchair-accessible, giving income-eligible residents a safe and comfortable environment in which to live. Located in New Jersey and North Carolina, on-site social services provide additional support to residents.

Staying Connected

The MS Association of America encourages clients to form new relationships, to share experiences and information and to enjoy improved well-being. One way of improving well-being is through awareness events, which include educational and motivational presentations and workshops. These provide information about MS, its symptoms, and available treatments, as well as news about helpful products or services.

MSAA's *Staying Connected* program also facilitates peer support and friendship through its *Networking Program*. This is an online community of individuals with MS and their carepartners who are interested in finding peer support and corresponding through e-mail exchange. The program's online directory is password-protected and available through MSAA's website.

THE MULTIPLE SCLEROSIS SOCIETY OF CANADA
175 Bloor Street East, Suite 700, Toronto, Ontario M4W 3R8, Canada; 416-922-6065; in Canada: 800-268-7582; www.mssociety.ca

The MS Society of Canada has a membership of 28,000, with seven regional divisions and nearly 120 chapters. The Head Office is in Toronto, and division offices are located in Dartmouth, Montreal, Toronto, Winnipeg, Regina, Edmonton, and Vancouver. It is the only national voluntary organization in Canada that supports both MS research and services for people with MS and their families. Its mission is "to be a leader in finding a cure for MS and enabling people affected by MS to enhance their quality of life." Annually, the Society provides over $10 million in research funding through pilot and operating grants, multi-center collaborative research grants, and personnel awards.

History

A small group of dedicated volunteers in Montreal founded the MS Society of Canada in 1948 after contact with the newly established National MS Society (USA). Its support of MS research began in 1949. The Society's headquarters remained in Montreal until the mid-1960s, when the offices moved to Toronto. Other advances came with the establishment of regional divisions, and there are now seven divisions across Canada, from coast to coast.

Client Services

The Society provides a wide variety of programs and services, available in both English and French, for those affected by MS. These include:

▶ **Information and Referral:** MS Society of Canada publications; www.msanswers.ca (a web-based MS-management resource); information and referrals over the phone, in person, or by e-mail
▶ **Education:** Conferences and workshops
▶ **Support:** Support and self-help groups; recreation and social programs
▶ **Advocacy:** Helping individuals with MS obtain needed services and resources
▶ **Funding:** Equipment purchase or loan programs; special assistance programs

Services vary across the country depending on the provincial government and community programs available, because the Society does not duplicate services available through other sources. The Society spends over $10 million annually on services and education programs for people with MS, family members, and others affected by MS.

Awareness Activities

The Society is firmly committed to informing Canadians about MS and how they can join the fight against it. The national office coordinates an overall public awareness campaign that is complemented by division and chapter activities.

Government Relations

The Society works with people who have MS, their families, and care providers to ensure that they have the opportunity to participate fully in all aspects of life. Volunteers across the country endeavor to change government policies at all levels, private industry practices, and public attitudes in ways that will positively benefit people with MS.

Fund-raising

The Society has total net revenues of over $30 million annually. The funds are used to support research, client services, public education, government relations, and volunteer resources. Most of this income comes from public donations, bequests, and special fund-raising programs conducted by the MS Society. The major fund-raising programs are the MS Carnation Campaign, the RONA MS Bike Tour, the MS Read-A-Thon, the MS WALK, the direct marketing program, and leadership giving.

MS Clinics

The Society works with a network of specialized MS clinics across the country. Clinic services vary, but most offer a wide range of services, delivered by a multi-disciplinary health care team. These services usually include expert diagnostic and treatment services for people with MS; clinical research, especially in the area of MS treatment options; and educational and support programs for people with MS and their families and caregivers.

Multiple Sclerosis Coalition Members (MSC)

Founded in 2005, the MSC is a collaborative network of independent MS organizations whose vision is to improve the quality of life for those affected by MS. As of 2009, the MSC membership includes the following organizations in addition to the **National MS Society** and the **MS Association of America**, all of which are dedicated to improving the quality of life for everyone affected by MS.

ACCELERATED CURE PROJECT FOR MULTIPLE SCLEROSIS

300 Fifth Avenue, Waltham, MA 02451 781-487-0008; www.acceleratedcure.org; info-web0209@acceleratedcure.org

This national nonprofit group is dedicated to curing MS by determining its causes. Its repository contains samples and data from people with MS and other demyelinating diseases. Samples are available to researchers who submit all data they generate back to the repository to be shared with others.

CONSORTIUM OF MULTIPLE SCLEROSIS CENTERS (CMSC)

359 Main Street, Suite A, Hackensack, NJ 07601; 201-487-1050; www.mscare.org

The mission of the CMSC is to be the preeminent professional organization for MS healthcare providers and researchers in North America, and a valued partner in the global MS community. Its core purpose is to maximize the ability of MS healthcare professionals to impact care of people who are affected by MS, thus improving their quality of life.

CAN DO MULTIPLE SCLEROSIS, FORMERLY THE HEUGA CENTER FOR MULTIPLE SCLEROSIS

27 Main Street, Suite 303, Edwards, CO 81632; 800-367-3101; 970-926-1290; www.mscando.org; info@mscando.org

Can Do MS, formerly The Heuga Center for Multiple Sclerosis, offers MS programs based on the philosophy of founder Jimmie Heuga, who believed that a person with a chronic disease can maintain optimal health. The Center provides wellness-centered programs for individuals with MS, their family members, and health care professionals. Programs include education, nutrition, mental well-being, and exercise, as well as learning specific, individualized life management skills and ways to integrate wellness activities into everyday life. The Center's programs help people set personal life goals as a focal point for reclaiming their lives, and then give them the strategies, confidence, and support to strive for those goals.

INTERNATIONAL ORGANIZATION OF MULTIPLE SCLEROSIS NURSES (IOMSN)

359 Main Street, Suite A, Hackensack, NJ 07601; 201-487-1050; www.iomsn.org

The mission of the IOMSN is the establishment and perpetuation of a specialized branch of nursing in MS; to establish standards of MS nursing care; to support MS nursing research; to educate the health care community about MS; and to disseminate this knowledge throughout the world.

MULTIPLE SCLEROSIS FOUNDATION (MSF)

6350 North Andrews Avenue, Fort Lauderdale, Florida 33309-2130; 800-225-6495; 954-776-6805; www.msfocus.org

This predominantly service-based organization focuses on helping people with MS maintain their health and well-being. It offers programs and support to enhance self-sufficiency and safety.

MSFRIENDS (MSFRIENDS INITIATIVE, THE VISIONWORKS FOUNDATION INC.)

2370 Market Street #347, San Francisco, CA 94114; 866-673-7436; www.msfriends.org

MSFriends is dedicated to improving the quality of life for people with MS, their families, and friends. It offers a 24/7 peer support telephone helpline in the continental U.S., staffed with volunteers who have MS. It offers the invaluable service of "Friends Helping Friends," immediate lifelines that offer MSFriends Guided Outreach to anyone, anywhere.

PARALYZED VETERANS OF AMERICA (PVA)

801 Eighteenth Street, NW, Washington, DC 20006; 800-424-8200; info@pva.org; www.pva.org

Paralyzed Veterans is a congressionally chartered veterans service organization that provides veterans' benefits services to service-connected and non-service connected veterans who have experienced a traumatic spinal cord injury or disease such as multiple sclerosis, ALS, or polio. It provides benefits counseling, information and referral services, and local networking resources for veterans and their families. Paralyzed Veterans also conducts programs in advocacy, architecture, clinical practice guidelines, education, governmental relations, medical services, publications, research, and sports.

UNITED SPINAL ASSOCIATION (USA)

75-20 Astoria Boulevard, Jackson Heights, New York 11370; 888-MSFOCUS, 718-803-3782; support@msfocus.org; www.unitedspinal.org

USA is dedicated to serving the needs of people with MS and other spinal cord disorders. It addresses a wide variety of issues including health care, home and community services, and medical equipment access. USA offers personalized consultations and many publications, including the *MS Quarterly Report.*

Appendix 1

Glossary

This glossary of terms commonly used in association with primary progressive multiple sclerosis (PPMS) is based on the more detailed MS glossary available on the National MS Society's website at: www.nationalmssociety.org/about-multiple-sclerosis/glossary/index.aspx.

Activities of daily living (ADLs): Any daily activity a person performs for self-care, work, homemaking, and leisure. The ability to perform ADLs is often used as a measure of ability/disability in MS.

Advance (medical) directive: Advance directives preserve a person's right to accept or reject a course of medical treatment, even if he or she becomes mentally or physically unable to communicate those wishes. The two basic forms are a living will and a health care proxy.

Ankle-foot orthosis (AFO): A brace worn on the lower leg and foot to support the ankle, correct foot drop, and promote correct heel-toe walking.

Antibody: A protein produced by certain cells of the immune system in response to bacteria, viruses, and other types of foreign antigens.

Antigen: Any substance that triggers the immune system to produce an antibody; the term generally refers to infectious or toxic substances.

Aspiration pneumonia: Inflammation of the lungs due to the inhalation of food particles or fluids.

Assistive devices: Any tools designed, fabricated, and/or adapted to assist a person in performing a particular task, such as a cane, walker, or shower chair.

Assistive technology: Tools, products, and devices that can make a particular function easier or possible to perform.

Atrophy: A wasting away or decrease in size of a cell, tissue, or organ of the body because of disease or lack of use.

Autoimmune disease: A disorder, such as MS, in which the body's immune system causes illness by mistakenly attacking healthy cells, organs, or tissues.

Axon: The extension or prolongation of a nerve cell (neuron) that conducts impulses to other nerve cells or muscles. Many axons in the CNS are covered with myelin.

B-cell: A type of lymphocyte (white blood cell) manufactured in the bone marrow that makes antibodies.

Blood–brain barrier: A cell layer around blood vessels in the brain and spinal cord that prevents potentially damaging substances and disease-causing organisms from passing out of the bloodstream into the CNS (brain and spinal cord). A break in the blood–brain barrier may underlie the disease process in MS.

Brainstem: That part of the CNS that contains the nerve centers for respiration and heart control. It extends from the base of the brain to the spinal cord.

Catheter: A hollow, flexible tube inserted through the urinary opening into the bladder to drain urine that cannot be excreted normally.

Central nervous system (CNS): The part of the nervous system that includes the brain, optic nerves, and spinal cord. The nerves that leave the spinal cord and go to the rest of the body make up the *peripheral nervous system.*

Cerebellum: A part of the brain situated above the brainstem that controls balance and coordination of movement.

Cerebrospinal fluid (CSF): A watery, colorless, clear fluid that bathes and protects the brain and spinal cord. The changes in CSF characteristic of MS can be detected with a lumbar puncture (spinal tap), a test sometimes used to help make the MS diagnosis.

Cerebrum: The large, upper part of the brain that acts as a master control system and is responsible for initiating thought and motor activity. Its two hemispheres are united by the corpus callosum and form the largest part of the CNS.

Chronic progressive MS: Former catch-all term for progressive forms of MS, now categorized as two separate forms of disease.

Clinical trial: A research study designed to answer specific questions about vaccines, new therapies, or new ways of using known treatments. Clinical trials are used to determine whether new drugs or treatments are both safe and effective.

Clonus: A sign of spasticity in which involuntary shaking or jerking of the leg occurs when the toe is placed on the floor with the knee slightly bent. The shaking is caused by repeated, rhythmic, reflex muscle contractions.

Cognition: High-level functions that include comprehension and use of speech, visual perception and construction, calculation ability, attention, memory, and executive functions such as planning, problem-solving, and self-monitoring.

Complementary and alternative therapy: A broad range of healing philosophies, approaches, and therapies, such as acupuncture and herbs, that conventional medicine does not commonly use to promote well-being or treat health conditions.

Computerized axial tomography (CT scan): A noninvasive diagnostic radiology technique that examines soft tissues of the body. A computer integrates X-ray scanned "slices" of the organ being examined into a cross-sectional picture.

Condom catheter: A tube connected to a thin, flexible sheath worn over the penis to allow drainage of urine into a collection system.

Constipation: A condition in which bowel movements happen less frequently than is normal, or the stool is small, hard, and difficult or painful to pass.

Contracture: A permanent shortening of the muscles and tendons adjacent to a joint that can result from severe, untreated spasticity, and that interferes with normal movement. If left untreated, the affected joint can become frozen in a flexed (bent) position.

Decubitus: An ulcer (sore) of the skin that results from pressure and lack of movement with advanced mobility issues. The ulcers occur most frequently in areas where bone lies directly under skin, such as the elbow, hip, or over the coccyx (tailbone).

Demyelination: A loss of myelin in the white matter of the CNS (brain, spinal cord).

Double-blind clinical study: A study in which none of the participants know who is taking the test drug and who is taking a control or *placebo* agent. This research design avoids inadvertent bias of the test results.

Evoked potentials (EPs): Recordings of the nervous system's electrical response to the stimulation of specific sensory pathways. Because demyelination results in a slowing of response time, EPs can demonstrate lesions along specific nerves, making this test useful in confirming the diagnosis of MS.

Expanded Disability Status Scale (EDSS): The EDSS summarizes the neurologic examination and provides a measure of overall disability. It is used for many reasons, including deciding future medical treatment, establishing rehabilitation goals, choosing participants for clinical trials, and measuring treatment outcomes.

Experimental autoimmune encephalomyelitis (formerly *experimental allergic encephalomyelitis*) **(EAE):** An autoimmune disease resembling MS that can be induced in some genetically susceptible research animals. Before testing on humans, a potential treatment for MS is often first tested on laboratory animals with EAE to determine the treatment's efficacy and safety.

Food and Drug Administration (FDA): The government agency responsible for enforcing regulations relating to the manufacture and sale of food, drugs, and cosmetics.

Foot drop: A condition of weakness in the muscles of the foot and ankle caused by poor nerve conduction, which interferes with the ability to flex the ankle and walk with a normal heel-toe pattern, causing the person to trip or lose balance.

Gadolinium-enhancing lesion: A lesion that appears on MRI following injection of the chemical compound gadolinium; it reveals a breakdown in the blood–brain barrier, indicating either a newly active lesion or the reactivation of an old one.

Helper T-lymphocytes: White blood cells that are a major contributor to the immune system's inflammatory response against myelin.

Immune system: A complex network of glands, tissues, circulating cells, and processes that protect the body by identifying and neutralizing abnormal or foreign substances.

Immune-mediated disease: A disease in which components of the immune system are responsible for the disease.

Impairment: Any loss or abnormality of psychological, physiologic, or anatomic structure or function resulting from injury or disease.

Indwelling catheter: A type of catheter that remains in the bladder either on a temporary or permanent basis.

Inflammation: Immunologic response of a tissue to injury, characterized by the mobilization of white blood cells and antibodies, swelling, and fluid accumulation.

Intermittent self-catheterization (ISC): A procedure in which a catheter is periodically inserted into the urinary opening to drain any urine from the bladder that remains after voiding.

Loftstrand crutch: A type of crutch with an attached holder for the forearm to provide extra support.

Lumbar puncture: A diagnostic procedure that uses a hollow needle to penetrate the spinal canal to remove cerebrospinal fluid, to test for changes in composition characteristic of MS.

Lymphocyte: A type of white blood cell; part of the immune system. Two main groups are B-lymphocytes, which originate in the bone marrow and produce antibodies, and T-lymphocytes, which are produced in the bone marrow and mature in the thymus.

Macrophage: A white blood cell that has the ability to ingest and destroy foreign substances such as bacteria and cell debris.

Magnetic resonance imaging (MRI): A diagnostic procedure that produces visual images of different body parts without the use of X-rays. MRI makes it possible to visualize and count lesions in the white matter of the brain and spinal cord.

Multiple Sclerosis Functional Composite (MSFC): A three-part, standardized, quantitative assessment instrument that measure leg function/ambulation (Timed 25-Foot Walk), arm/hand function (Nine-Hole

Peg Test), and cognitive function (Paced Auditory Serial Addition Test [PASAT]).

Myelin: The soft, white coating of nerve fibers in the CNS, composed of lipids (fats) and protein. Myelin serves as insulation and aids efficient nerve fiber conduction. Nerve fiber conduction is faulty or absent when myelin is damaged in MS.

Myelin basic protein (MBP): One of several proteins associated with the myelin of the CNS, which may be found in higher than normal concentrations in the cerebrospinal fluid of individuals with MS and other diseases that damage myelin.

Nerve: A bundle of nerve fibers (axons) that are either *afferent* (leading toward the brain and involved in the perception of sensory stimuli of the skin, joints, muscles, and inner organs), or *efferent* (leading away from the brain and mediating contractions of muscles or organs).

Nervous system: Includes all neural structures in the body. The *central nervous system* includes the brain, spinal cord, and optic nerves; the *peripheral nervous system* includes nerves throughout the body.

Neurogenic bladder: Bladder dysfunction associated with malfunction in the spinal cord. Symptoms include urinary urgency, frequency, hesitancy, nocturia, and incontinence.

Occupational therapist (OT): OTs assess essential activities of everyday living, including dressing, bathing, grooming, meal preparation, writing, and driving.

Off-label use: A drug prescribed for conditions other than those approved by the FDA.

Oligoclonal bands: A diagnostic sign that indicates abnormal levels of certain antibodies in the cerebrospinal fluid; they are seen in approximately 90 percent of people with MS.

Oligodendrocyte: A type of cell in the CNS that is responsible for making and supporting myelin.

Optic atrophy: A wasting of the optic disc that results from partial or complete degeneration of optic nerve fibers; it is associated with loss of visual acuity.

Orthotic: Also called *orthosis*; a mechanical appliance such as a leg brace or splint that is specially designed to control, correct, or compensate for impaired limb function.

Orthotist: A person skilled in making mechanical appliances (orthotics) such as leg braces or splints that help support limb function.

Osteoporosis: Decalcification of the bones, which can result from the lack of mobility experienced by wheelchair-bound individuals.

Physiatrist: Physicians who specialize in physical medicine and rehabilitation, including the diagnosis and management of musculoskeletal injuries and pain syndromes, electrodiagnostic medicine (e.g., electromyography), and the rehabilitation of severe impairments, including those caused by neurologic disease or injury.

Physical therapist (PT): PTs evaluate and improve movement and function of the body, with particular attention to physical mobility, balance, posture, fatigue, and pain.

Placebo: An inactive, nondrug compound that looks like the test drug. It is administered to control group subjects in double-blind clinical trials as a way of assessing the benefits and liabilities of the test drug taken by experimental group subjects.

Plaque: An area of inflamed or demyelinated CNS tissue. A plaque (or lesion), which can vary from a few millimeters to a few centimeters in diameter, generally contains white blood cells and other cells involved in brain inflammation.

Primary progressive MS (PPMS): A form of MS characterized by disease progression from onset, without relapses and remissions.

Progressive relapsing MS (PRMS): A form of MS with disease progression from the beginning, but with clear, acute relapses, with or without full recovery. Periods between relapses are characterized by continuing progression.

Rehabilitation: Rehabilitation in MS involves multidisciplinary strategies to promote functional independence, prevent unnecessary complications, and enhance overall quality of life. Its goal is to help the person recover and/or maintain the highest possible level of function and potential, given any limitations that exist.

Relapsing remitting MS: A form of MS characterized by clearly defined, acute attacks with full or partial recovery and no disease progression between attacks.

Secondary progressive MS: A form of MS that initially is relapsing remitting and then becomes progressive, possibly with an occasional relapse and minor remission.

Sign: An objective physical problem or abnormality identified by the physician during the neurologic examination. Neurologic signs may differ significantly from the symptoms reported by the patient because they are identifiable only with specific tests and might cause no overt symptoms.

Spasticity: An abnormal increase in muscle tone, shown as a spring-like resistance to moving or being moved.

Speech/language pathologist: Specialists in the diagnosis and treatment of speech, swallowing, and cognitive-communication disorders.

Symptom: A subjectively perceived problem or complaint reported by the patient.

T1 and T2 Lesions: T1 images show "black holes," which are believed to indicate areas of permanent damage to axons and other CNS components. T2-weighted MRI scans provide information about disease *burden* or *lesion load*—the total amount of current damage.

T-cell: A lymphocyte (white blood cell) that develops in the bone marrow, matures in the thymus, and works as part of the immune system in the body.

Transcutaneous electric nerve stimulation (TENS): A nonaddictive and noninvasive method of pain control that applies electric impulses to nerve endings via electrodes that are attached to a stimulator by flexible wires and placed on the skin. The electric impulses block the transmission of pain signals to the brain.

Visual evoked potential (VEP): A test in which the brain's electrical activity is measured in response to visual stimuli. Demyelination slows response time. It can confirm the presence of a suspected brain lesion and detect unsuspected lesions that have not produced symptoms; it is extremely useful in diagnosing MS.

Vocational rehabilitation (VR): A program of services that enable people with disabilities to become or remain employed. Programs typically evaluate the disability and need for adaptive equipment or mobility aids, and provide vocational guidance, training, job-placement, and follow-up.

White matter: The part of the brain that contains myelin-coated nerve fibers—and therefore appears white—in contrast to the cortex of the brain, which contains nerve cell bodies and appears gray.

Appendix 2

Resources

GENERAL RESOURCES

Books

Holland NJ, Halper J. *Multiple Sclerosis: A Self-Care Guide to Wellness*, 2nd Ed. New York: Demos Medical Publishing, 2005.

Kalb R, ed. *Multiple Sclerosis: The Questions You Have; The Answers You Need*, 4th Ed. New York: Demos Medical Publishing, 2008.

Kalb R, Holland NJ, Giesser B. *Multiple Sclerosis for Dummies*. New York: Wiley, 2007.

Information Resources

Medline Plus; www.medlineplus.gov is a service of the National Library of Medicine and the National Institutes of Health that provides health news, drug information, clinical trials listing, a medical encyclopedia, a medical dictionary, and links to other databases and resources.

National Multiple Sclerosis Society. NMSS Publications can be accessed at: www.nationalMSsocietyorg/brochures.

Multiple Sclerosis Association of America. Publications can be accessed at: www.msassociation.org/publications.

Department of Veterans Affairs (VA). 800-827-1000; www.va.gov. The VA provides a wide range of benefits and services to those who have served in the armed forces, their dependents, benefici-

aries of deceased veterans, and dependent children of veterans
with disabilities.

National Health Information Center, P.O. Box 1133, Washington,
D.C. 20013; 800-336-4797; www.health.gov/nhic. The Center
maintains a library and a database of health-related organizations,
and provides referrals related to health issues for consumers and
professionals.

National Rehabilitation Information Center (NARIC). 800-346-2742
or 301-459-5900; www.naric.com. NARIC is a library and information center on disability and rehabilitation funded by the National
Institute on Disability and Rehabilitation Research (NIDRR).

Multiple Sclerosis International Federation (MSIF). +44 (0) 207-
620-1911; www.msif.org/. This international organization links
the activities of MS societies worldwide. Its website includes access
to numerous publications.

RESOURCES BY CHAPTER

In addition to materials that can be downloaded from the National
MS Society and the MS Association of America websites, publications from both organizations can be requested by phone. National
MS Society publications are available free of charge in hard copy
from your local chapter, at: 800-FIGHT-MS (800-344-4867). Many
chapters have a lending library and also can provide copies of book
publications. The MS Association of America's articles and publications can be ordered free of charge by calling 800-532-7667; publications and DVD copies of the online MSi videos can be borrowed
from MSAA's free Lending Library.

Chapter 3. Research and Clinical Trials

Cutter G, Aban A. *The Confusing World of Clinical Trials: A Guide for
Patients and Families.* View or download at: www.msassociation.org/
publications/monograph/ct/.

Multiple Sclerosis Association of America. MSi on-demand video, *A
Closer Look at MS Research—2009 and Beyond.* Access at: www.
msassociation.org/programs/videos/closerlook_research2009.asp.

National MS Society. *Clinical Trial Resources from the National MS Society.* Access at: www.nationalmssociety.org/research/clinical-trials/clinical-trial-resources/index.aspx.

National MS Society. *My Life, My MS, My Decision.* This four-part video contains a section on clinical trials, with a section that focuses on making the decision whether to enter a clinical trial. Access at: www.nationalmssociety.org/multimedia-library/videos

Norris C, Courtney SW. *Making Sense of MS Terminology: A Guide to Understanding Medical Terms and Procedures for Individuals with MS.* View or download at: www.msassociation.org/publications/summer07/health.asp.

Richert J, Schneider DM. *Research Directions in Multiple Sclerosis.* This booklet can be downloaded at: www.nationalmssociety.org/search-results/index.aspx?pageindex=0&pagesize=20&keywords=Richert percent2C+Research+brochure.

Schneider DM. *MS Research Update 2009.* View or download at: www.msassociation.org/publications/summer09/cover.story.asp.

Resources for Locating Clinical Trials

Information about trials that are recruiting people with MS can be downloaded at: www.nationalmssociety.org/site/PageServer?pagename=HOM_RES_research_trialsrecruiting.

National MS Society. *Clinical Trials in MS 2009*, a National MS Society booklet, can be downloaded at: www.nationalmssociety.org/ClinicalTrials. This site also contains other useful information on clinical trials.

MSAA's Clinical Trials Resource Center is at www.msaassociation.org/programs/cti/.

Chapter 4. An Overview of PPMS Management: How Does Rehabilitation Maintain and Improve Function?

National MS Society. *Managing MS Through Rehabilitation.* This brochure can be downloaded from: www.nationalmssociety.org/search-results/index.aspx?pageindex=0&pagesize=20&keywords=Managing+MS+Through+Rehabilitation&x=32&y=12.

Courtney SW, Lucuski LA. *The Benefits of Rehabilitation.* View or download at: www.msassociation.org/publications/winter04/cover.asp.

Chapter 5. Symptom Management: Treatment Options

Both the National MS Society and the MS Association of America have articles and brochures dealing with specific MS symptoms. Simply enter the symptom into the "Search" field to view and/or download from their respective websites.

Bowling AC. *Complementary and Alternative Medicine and Multiple Sclerosis*, 2nd ed. Demos Medical Publishing, 2007.

Cooling. For information about the potential benefits of cooling, as well as the MS Association's Cooling Equipment Distribution program, visit www.msassociation.org/programs/cooling/ or call 800-532-7667.

Courtney SW. *Heat Sensitivity* can be viewed or downloaded at: www.msassociation.org/publications/summer05/symptom.asp.

Multiple Sclerosis Association of America. The MSi on-demand video, *A Closer Look at MS and Complementary and Alternative Medicine*, can be viewed at: www.msassociation.org/programs/videos/closerlook5.asp.

Multiple Sclerosis Association of America. Multiple Sclerosis Information (MSi) on-demand video, *A Closer Look at Multiple Sclerosis Symptoms—Part I*, can be viewed at: www.msassociation.org/programs/videos/closerlook1.asp; the MSi on-demand video, *The Art of Symptom Management – MS in the 21st Century*, can be viewed at www.msassociation.org/programs/videos/ and selecting this title.

Multiple Sclerosis Association of America. *Understanding Integrative Medicine*. View or download at: www.msassociation.org/publications/winter07/.

Peterman Schwarz S. *Keeping Your Cool* can be viewed or downloaded at: www.msassociation.org/publications/summer07/symptom.asp.

Schapiro R. *Managing the Symptoms of Multiple Sclerosis*, 5th ed. New York: Demos Medical Publishing, 2007.

Schneider DM. *Symptom Management Update*. View or download at: www.msassociation.org/publications/winter09/cover.story.asp.

Stewart TM, Bowling AC. *Thinking About Complementary and Alternative Medicine? An Introduction for People with MS on How to Find and Evaluate Claims About Complementary and Alternative Medicine*. View or download at: www.msassociation.org/publications/monograph/cam/.

Chapter 6. Technology and Adaptations That Can Make Life with PPMS Easier to Manage

Books

Holland NJ, Halper J. *Multiple Sclerosis: A Self-Care Guide to Wellness*, 2nd ed. New York: Demos Medical Publishing, 2005.

Peterman Schwarz S. *Multiple Sclerosis: 300 Tips for Making Life Easier*, 2nd ed. New York: Demos Medical Publishing, 2006.

General Resources

Many catalogs and websites that deal with helpful products for people with disabilities can be found at: www.google.com/ search?sourceid=navclient&ie=UTF-8&rlz=1T4ADBR_ enUS296US296&q=disability+products+catalogs. Two that might be especially useful are www.alimed.com and www.maxiaids.com; www.homecontrols.com is a catalog supplier of home automation devices.

For information about the Multiple Sclerosis Association of America's Equipment Distribution program, visit www.msassociation.org/ programs/equipment/ or call 800-532-7667.

ABLEDATA; 800-227-0216. Access at: www.abledata.com/abledata. This site provides information on assistive technology and rehabilitation equipment available from domestic and international sources.

Meeting Life's Challenges, LLC. *Making Life Easier for People with Chronic Illness, Disability, or Age-related Limitations*. Access at: http://meetinglifeschallenges.com/index.php. Shelley Peterman Schwarz' site has links to products, resources, services, books, and programs that provide support, encouragement, and strategies for living with MS.

Driving

The National Mobility Equipment Dealers Association (NMEDA). Accessing www.nmeda.org connects people with disabilities to companies that can help meet their transportation needs.

Peterman Schwarz S. *The Driving Question: Do the Symptoms of MS Interfere with Your Driving?* View or download at: www.msassociation.org/publications/fall06/driving.question.asp.

Tromp van Holst F, Valois T. Driving and Other Transportation Issues. In: Holland NJ, Halper J, eds. *Multiple Sclerosis: A Self-Care Guide to Wellness*. New York: Demos Medical Publishing, 2005.

Home Accessibility

Davies TD, Lopez CP. Making Your Home Safe and More Accessible. In: Holland NJ, Halper J, eds. *Multiple Sclerosis: A Self-Care Guide to Wellness*. New York: Demos Medical Publishing, 2005.

Davies TD, Lopez CP. *Accessible Home Design: Architectural Solutions for the Wheelchair User*. Washington DC: Paralyzed Veterans of America, 2006.

Multiple Sclerosis Association of America. The MSi on-demand video, *Making Your Home Work for You—Improving Home Safety and Accessibility*, can be viewed at: www.msassociation.org/programs/videos/closerlook_work.asp.

www.nationalMSsociety.org/MSLearnOnline has a series of four videos hosted by Shelley Peterman Schwarz on home adaptations for specific rooms.

Computer Access

Bruce C. *Minimizing the Digital Divide for Individuals with MS: A three-part series on strategies, equipment, and software to increase computer accessibility*. View or download at: www.msassociation.org/publications/fall04/digital.asp; www.msassociation.org/publications/winter05/digital.asp; www.msassociation.org/publications/spring05/digital. asp.

Chapter 7. Wellness and Primary Progressive Multiple Sclerosis: An Attainable Goal

General Health and Wellness

Brochures on a wide range of wellness-related topics can be downloaded at: www.nationalmssociety.org/site/PageServer?pagename=HOM_LIB.

Courtney SW. *Healthcare Beyond MS*. View or download at: www.msassociation.org/publications/winter05/ beyondms.asp.

Courtney SW. *Partners in Wellness: The Importance of a Positive Doctor–Patient Relationship*. View or download at: www.msassociation.org/publications/spring08/cover.story.asp.

http://www.nationalmssociety.org/living-with-multiple-sclerosis/
getting-the-care-you-need/my-life-my-ms-my-decisions/index
.aspx

Holland NJ, Halper J. *Multiple Sclerosis: A Self-Care Guide to Wellness.*
New York: Demos Medical Publishing, 2005.

Can Do MS, formerly The Heuga Center for Multiple Sclerosis, is a
national nonprofit organization and an innovative provider of
lifestyle empowerment programs for people with MS and their
support partners. Access at: www.mscando.org.

National MS Society. *Preventive Care Recommendations for Adults
with MS* is a chart detailing the medical tests, vaccinations, and
general health and safety rules recommended for all adults with
MS. Access at: www.nationalmssociety.org/site/Search?query=
Preventive+Care+Recommendations+for+Adults+with+MS.

Nutrition and Weight Management

Embry A. *Nutritional Factors and Multiple Sclerosis.* View or download
this three-part series at: www.msassociation.org/publications/
winter04/health.asp; www.msassociation.org/publications/summer
04/health.asp; and www.msassociation.org/publications/fall04/
health.asp.

Hunsberger MB. *Health and Wellness: Nutritional Tips for Individuals
with MS.* Viewed or download at: www.msassociation.org/
publications/summer08/health.asp.

Hunsberger MB. *Weight Management and MS.* View or download at:
www.msassociation.org/publications/spring08/symptom.asp.

Exercise

The National MS Society's website, www.nationalmssociety.org, has
many articles on specific forms of exercise, such as aquatics, yoga,
and tai-chi; simply enter the appropriate term into the "Search" field.

Multiple Sclerosis Association of America. MSi on-demand video, *A
Closer Look at The Benefits of Exercise,* can be viewed at: www.
msassociation.org/programs/videos/closerlook_benefits.exercise.asp.

Chapter 8. Emotional and Quality-of-Life Issues

Stress

Courtney SW, Franco M. *Imagine the Possibilities: An Introduction to
Guided Imagery and Its Potential Benefits for Individuals with MS.*

View or download at: www.msassociation.org/publications/
winter08/cover.story.asp.

LaRocca NG. *Emotional Changes and the Role of Stress*. In: Kalb R.
Multiple Sclerosis: The Questions You Have; The Answers You Need,
Fourth Edition. New York: Demos Medical Publishing, 2008.

Multiple Sclerosis Association of America. *A Closer Look at Managing
Stress and MS*, an MSi on-demand video, can be viewed at:
www.msassociation.org/programs/videos/closerlook9.asp.

National MS Society. *Taming Stress in Multiple Sclerosis*. Available at:
www.nationalmssociety.org/site/PageServer?pagename=HOM_
LIB_brochures_tamingstress1.

Emotional Issues

*Multiple Sclerosis and Your Emotions: How to Manage Some of the
Emotional Challenges Created by MS* is at: http://www.nationalms
society.org/multimedia-library/brochures/staying-well/
index.aspx. Click on the file Multiple Sclerosis and Your Emotions
to download.

Multiple Sclerosis Association of America. The MSi on-demand
video *A Closer Look at the Emotional Impact of MS* can be viewed
at: www.msassociation.org/programs/videos/closerlook8.asp.

Cognition

Courtney SW. *Strategies to Help with Cognitive Problems*. View or
download at: www.msassociation.org/publications/spring06/
symptom.awareness.asp.

LaRocca N, Kalb R. *Multiple Sclerosis: Understanding the Cognitive
Challenges*. New York: Demos Medical Publishing, 2006.

Depression

Courtney SW. *Dealing With Depression*. View or download at:
www.msassociation.org/publications/fall05/symptom.asp.

National MS Society. *Depression and Multiple Sclerosis*. Download at:
www.nationalmssociety.org/site/PageServer?pagename=HOM_
LIB_brochures_on_depression

Shadday A. *Understanding and Treating Depression in Multiple
Sclerosis: Recognizing the Symptoms and Learning the Solutions*.
View or download at: www.msassociation.org/publications/
depression/MSAA.Depression.0507.pdf.

Chapter 9. Family and Social Issues

Kalb RC. *Multiple Sclerosis: A Guide for Families*, 3rd ed. New York: Demos Medical Publishing, 2006.

Intimacy

Courtney SW. *Rediscovering Intimacy*. View or download at: www.msassociation.org/publications/fall04/ redint.asp.

Foley F. Sexuality and Intimacy in Multiple Sclerosis. In: Kalb RC, ed. *Multiple Sclerosis: A Guide for Families*, 3rd ed. New York: Demos Medical Publishing, 2006.

Kroll K, Levy E. *Enabling Romance: A Guide to Love, Sex, and Relationships for People with Disabilities (and the People Who Care About Them)*. Baltimore: No Limits Communications, 2001.

Multiple Sclerosis Association of America. The MSi on-demand video, *A Closer Look at Intimacy and MS*, can be viewed at: www.msassociation.org/programs/videos/closerlook4.asp.

National MS Society. *Intimacy and Sexuality in MS*. Download at: www.nationalmssociety.org/search-results/index.aspx?pageindex =0&pagesize=20&keywords=Intimacy+and+Sexuality+in+MS

National MS Society. The webcasts *Positive Relationships and Together in the MS Journey* can be viewed at: www.nationalmssociety. org/MSLearnOnline.

Parenting

Courtney SW. *Mommy's Story: An Introduction for Younger Children to Learn About a Parent's MS*. View or download at: www.msassociation.org/PDFs/Mommy's_Story_09.pdf.

Crawford P, Miller D. Parenting Issues. In: Kalb RC. *Multiple Sclerosis: A Guide for Families*, 3rd ed. New York: Demos Medical Publishing, 2006.

National MS Society Resources for Children: *Keep S'myelin* newsletter for children whose parents have MS.

National MS Society. *Timmy's Journey to Understanding MS*. DVD is available from the National MS Society. Contact NMSS at: www.nationalMSsocietyorg/brochures.

Rogers J. *The Disabled Woman's Guide to Pregnancy and Birth*. New York: Demos Medical Publishing, 2006.

Through the Looking Glass: National Research and Training Center on Families of Adults with Disabilities; 800-644-2666;

www.lookingglass.org. Publications include Adaptive Parenting: Idea Book I.

Friends and Networking

The MS Association of America's Networking program connects individuals with MS, as well as their carepartners, with one another via e-mail. For more information, visit support.msassociation.org/Networking.

Travel

The American Automobile Association (AAA) has materials for people with disabilities; contact them for help with trip planning. Call your local branch office.

Accessible Journeys; 800-846-4537, 610-521-0339 arranges travel for mobility-impaired travelers. Access at: www.disabilitytravel.com/

Courtney SW. *Planning Your Vacation.* Call MSAA at 800-225-6495; 954-776-6805 to order a free copy.

Harrington C. *101 Accessible Vacations: Travel Ideas for Wheelers and Slow Walkers.* New York: Demos Medical Publishing, 2008.

Harrington C. *Barrier-Free Travel: A Nuts and Bolts Guide for Wheelers and Slow Walkers.* New York: Demos Medical Publishing, 2005.

Harrington C. *There Is Room at the Inn: Inns and B&Bs for Wheelers and Slow Walkers.* New York: Demos Medical Publishing, 2006.

National Library Service for the Blind and Physically Handicapped. *Information for Handicapped Travelers.* Available free of charge. Contact at: 800-424-8567; 202-707-5100; www.loc.gov/nls/; enls@loc.gov.

National Parks Service. Access at: www.nps.gov.

Norris C. *Travel the Easy Way . . . Just Pack Your Bags and Go!* View or download at: www.msassociation.org/publications/summer05/travel.asp.

Chapter 10. Carepartner Support and Resources

Books and Articles

Banister KR. *The Personal Care Attendant Guide: The Art of Finding, Keeping, or Being One.* New York: Demos Medical Publishing, 2007.

Courtney SW. *Caring for a Loved One.* View or download at: www.msassociation.org/publications/spring04/cover.asp.

Frankel D, Cavallo P. Obtaining Personal Assistance. In: Holland NJ, Halper J, eds. *Multiple Sclerosis: A Self-Care Guide to Wellness.* New York: Demos Medical Publishing, New York, 2005.

Meyer MM, Derr P, with the National MS Society. *The Comfort of Home Multiple Sclerosis Edition: An Illustrated Step-by-Step Guide for Multiple Sclerosis Caregivers.* Portland OR: Care Trust Publishing, 2006.

Miller D, Crawford P. The Caregiving Relationship. In: Kalb R, ed. *Multiple Sclerosis: A Guide for Families.* New York: Demos Medical Publishing, 2006.

Northrop DE, Frankel D. *Caring for Loved Ones with Advanced MS: A Guide for Families.* National MS Society

Websites

www.caregiving.com offers a monthly newsletter, *Spotlight on Caregiving*, that focuses on lifestyle changes brought on by caregiving. Its program, *The School of You*, offers classes focusing on caregiver stress, a weekly tips segment, and a support center.

www.fi avolunteers.org provides connection to volunteers offering nonmedical assistance.

www.alznyc.org/caregivers/homecare.asp#choose. This site provides excellent guidelines to choosing home care providers.

www.alznyc.org. The web page of the New York chapter of the Alzheimer's Association has practical, hands-on information and resources for caregiving.

Organizations for Caregivers

MedicAlert Foundation International; www.medicalert.org.

The National Family Caregivers Association (NFCA); www.nfcacares.org; 800-896-3650 provides a quarterly newsletter, a resource guide, and acts as an information clearinghouse.

The Well Spouse Association; 800-838-0879; www.wellspouse.org; is an emotional support network for people with a chronically ill partner.

Chapter 11. Economic Issues

General Resources

The National MS Society's website is an excellent source of detailed information about employment issues. See www.nationalmssociety.org/living-with-multiple-sclerosis/employment/index.aspx.

Cooper LD. Life Planning: Financial and Legal Considerations for Families Living with MS. In: Kalb R., ed. *Multiple Sclerosis: A Guide for Families.* New York: Demos Medical Publishing, 2006.

Financial Planning

Adapting: Financial Planning for a Life with Multiple Sclerosis addresses financial organization, planning, insurance options, employment concerns, and benefit issues important to people with PPMS and their families. Call the National MS Society at 800-FIGHT-MS or the Paralyzed Veterans of America Distribution Center at: 888-860-7244; you can also download or view the booklet in PDF format at: www.national mssociety.org/living-with-multiple-sclerosis/insurance-and-money-matters/financial-planning/index.aspx.

Courtney SW, Foy TD. *The Basics of Financial Planning: Seeking Financial Security for the Years Ahead.* View or download at www.msassociation.org/publications/spring06/basics.asp.

The National MS Society Collaborative Program with Financial Education Partners provides pro bono counsel by members of the Society of Financial Service Professionals. Call the National MS Society for details.

Insurance

Joyner AR, Courtney SW. *Ensuring Your Future: Selecting Insurance for You and Your Family's Financial Security.* View or download at: www.msassociation.org/publications/summer04/cover.asp.

Northrop DE, Cooper SE, Calder K. *Health Insurance Resources: A Guide for People with Chronic Disease and Disability,* 2nd ed. New York: Demos Medical Publishing, 2007.

Legal Assistance

National Academy of Elderlaw Attorneys, www.naela.org; or the Special Needs Alliance, www.specialneedsalliance.com can provide caregivers with referrals to local resources for creating special needs trusts.

Norris C. *Planning For the Future: The Importance of Advance Directives.* View or download at: www.msassociation.org/publications/fall05/planning.asp.

Perkins LE, Perkins SD. Multiple Sclerosis: *Your Legal Rights*, 3rd ed. New York: Demos Medical Publishing, 2008.

Shenkman MM. *Estate Planning for People with a Chronic Condition or Disability*. New York: Demos Medical Publishing, 2008.

Employment

A Closer Look at Employment and MS, www.msassociation. org/programs/videos/closerlook_employment.asp.

Multiple Sclerosis Association of America. Breaking Up Is Hard To Do: When Your Job Gets the Better of You. View or download at: www.msassociation.org/publications/winter07/health.asp.

Multiple Sclerosis Association of America. *Employment Strategies*. View or download at: www.msassociation.org/publications/ spring05/employmentstrategies.asp.

Operation Job Match is a National MS Society program that helps people with disabilities make decisions about returning to the workforce, retaining current employment, or changing to another job or career. Access at: www.nationalmssociety.org/chapters/ DCW/programs—services/employment/index.aspx.

President's Committee on Employment of People with Disabilities; www.usccr.gov/pubs/crd/federal/pcepd.htm; 800-526-7234; 202-376-6200 publishes employment-related brochures for individuals with disabilities and their employers, and provides a Job Accommodation Network.

Social Security Disability Benefits

Social Security Administration; 800-772-1213; www.ssa.gov. To apply for social security benefits based on disability, call this office or visit your local social security branch office.

Medicare information is available at: www.medicare.com.

Additional information available from the National MS Society is available at: www.nationalMS society.org/SSDI.

A Closer Look at Understanding Disability Benefits www. msassociation.org/programs/videos/closerlook_disability.asp.

Center for Medicare & Medicaid Services (CMS); www.cms.gov, provides numbers for many different individuals and categories of questions, or consult with your National MS Society chapter. The Nursing Home Compare feature on this government website evaluates nursing homes around the country in terms of several key indicators.

National MS Society. *Social Security Disability Benefits: A Guide for People Living with Multiple Sclerosis.* Access at: www. nationalmssociety.org.

National MS Society. *Social Security Disability Benefits for People Living with Multiple Sclerosis: A Guide for Professionals.* Access at: www.nationalmssociety.org.

NOSSCR, the National Organization of Social Security Claimants' Representatives, www.nosscr.org, is an association of attorneys and other advocates who represent Social Security and Supplemental Security Income claimants.

Personal Assistance

Banister KR. *The Personal Care Attendant Guide: The Art of Finding, Keeping, or Being One.* New York: Demos Medical Publishing, 2007.

Long-term Care Providers

The Boston Home; 617-825-3905 serves adults with advanced MS and other progressive neurologic diseases, on both a residential and outpatient basis.

Inglis House; 2600 Belmont Avenue, Philadelphia, PA 19131; 215-878-5600; www.inglis.org. A skilled nursing care facility for adults with physical disabilities. Services include long-term, rehabilitative medical and nursing care; physical, occupational and speech therapies; and social enrichment programs including computer and education therapy, vocational rehabilitation, therapeutic recreation and religious programs.

The Centers for Independent Living is a network of centers that offer technical advice, training, and advocacy to promote people with disabilities remaining in their homes. To locate a nearby center, go to www.ncil.org.

Index

Notes

NOTES

NOTES

NOTES